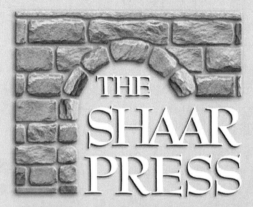

THE SHAAR PRESS

THE JUDAICA IMPRINT
FOR THOUGHTFUL PEOPLE

Tzipi Caton

MIRACLE

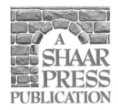

A SHAAR
PRESS
PUBLICATION

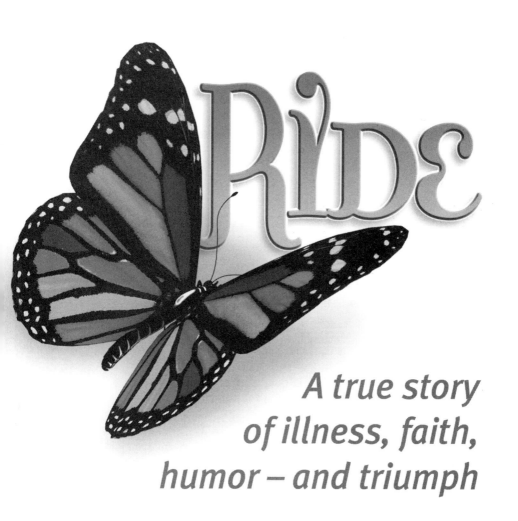

RiDE

**A true story
of illness, faith,
humor – and triumph**

Published by **SHAAR PRESS**
Distributed by MESORAH PUBLICATIONS, LTD.
4401 Second Avenue / Brooklyn, N.Y 11232 / (718) 921-9000 / www.artscroll.com

Distributed in Israel by SIFRIATI / A. GITLER
6 Hayarkon Street / Bnei Brak 51127

Distributed in Europe by LEHMANNS
Unit E, Viking Business Park, Rolling Mill Road / Jarrow, Tyne and Wear, NE32 3DP/ England

Distributed in Australia and New Zealand by GOLDS WORLD OF JUDAICA
3-13 William Street / Balaclava, Melbourne 3183 / Victoria Australia

Distributed in South Africa by KOLLEL BOOKSHOP
Ivy Common, 105 William Road / Norwood 2192, Johannesburg, South Africa

ISBN 10: 1-4226-0757-7 / ISBN 13: 978-1-4226-0757-2 (H/C)

Printed in the United States of America by Noble Book Press
Custom bound by Sefercraft, Inc. / 4401 Second Avenue / Brooklyn N.Y. 11232

For

Dr. Michael Harris

who treats those in his care

not just as patients,

but as people.

Table of Contents

Preface

By Michael B. Harris, M.D.

How does it feel to have your adolescence interrupted by a disease that robs you of your freedom, childhood dreams, body image and dignity? In *Miracle Ride*, Tzipi Caton's diary of her experiences with Hodgkin's disease, we find out. What began as a therapeutic exercise that allowed her to vent with pen and paper, turned into an insightful description of her journey through a twisted, uncharted tunnel full of obstacles and detours. Tzipi describes with sardonic wit and utter honesty the impact that the diagnosis and treatment of a life-threatening illness had on her, her family, her friends, and the community she lives in.

Tzipi is my patient. I remember well the adolescent I met on the cusp of womanhood and the woman who emerged after treatment was completed. Yet, as well as I thought I knew her, her diary taught me how much I did not know. The vignettes that fill her memoir speak of a young woman who realized the reality of her altered adolescence, unattained dreams, forever changed relationships, perceptions of community, and emotional and physical pain.

The question that Tzipi asked herself is, "How do I get through this and come out intact?" She decided to be open, feisty, unyielding, and to seize moments of happiness to gird her against the many moments of challenge. She sought help from all — whether medical staff, family, friends, or understanding adults. To become reclusive she realized was a self-destructive approach. Finally, and evident throughout her writings, was a deep faith in G-d's divine plan, "... because He's the one calling all the shots." But let's not misunderstand, Tzipi was not one to sit back for the ride and trust solely in G-d; she fought for everything she held dear — her life, her values, and her relationships.

Tzipi emerged victorious with a deeper understanding of her individuality, character traits, and faith. *Miracle Ride* is an excellent resource that teaches patients how to face a potentially deadly illness, and their families, friends, and the public how to interact with understanding, empathy, and support. *Miracle Ride* is a memoir that should be read by all.

Michael B. Harris, M.D.
Director, Tomorrow's Children's Institute
Joseph M. Sanzari Children's Hospital
Hackensack University Medical Center
Professor of Pediatrics
UMDNJ — New Jersey Medical School and
Touro University College of Medicine

Foreword

Going Along for the Ride: A Mother's Note

by Tzipi's Mother

So what is it like to be parents of a child with cancer? There is the anguish of seeing a child suffer, even though you trust that everything being done for her is only for the best. There is the agony of the decision-making: Which hospital? Which doctor? What treatment? Which highway to take to the emergency room during rush hour? There is the constant vigilance to symptoms that may be a sign of infection. There is the struggle to make sure that the rest of the family is taken care of. And there is the prolonged tiredness that comes from being in the hospital and doing absolutely nothing.

I would not be saying the truth if I didn't admit to how difficult it is to see your child suffer so deeply. No one should ever have to endure the sight of their suffering child and be able to say only, "But this is for your own good." It is a feeling of utter helplessness to see the glassy-eyed look of chemo descend on your child's face and know it's only the beginning of a long cycle.

Our children are our pride and joy, the reason for us to go on. The thought that something bad is happening to a person who is in reality an extension of oneself brings intense pain. I would even venture to say that the pain of a child is felt as if it were the parent's own.

Ironically, although we definitely experienced all of the above, I recall that period mostly as one of warmth and caring. There isn't and never was any bitterness about "Why us," "Why now." Only a perception of Divine Design remains with me from that time. Hashem held our hand and guided us from the diagnosis to the *chupah* and beyond. It was obvious to us from the start that we were being guided from Above. One day, as we were waiting for yet another test, we listed off to each other all the *hashgachah pratis* incidents that we had experienced. It was like a neon sign flashing in Heaven saying, "You must go through this now, but I will show you that you are not alone." For instance, it always struck me as strange that I reacted so quickly to my daughter's initial call that she felt a bump in her neck. I am very laid back when it comes to any complaints about minor aches and pains. Ordinarily I would have just said to wait a few days (or weeks) and see what develops.

All that being said, it was never far from my mind that we were the lucky ones. There were so many out there who were not given the option to have their cancers diagnosed at an early stage. I recall a precious four-year-old girl whose rash on her foot was misdiagnosed and now she is paralyzed, and another teenager with Hodgkin's who caught it at its final stages and didn't make it, or a sweet princess who relapsed after a bone marrow transplant and left us a few months later. Those were all kids in our ward. These were kids my daughter tied bandannas with, took chemo with, and whom she held hands with as she faced her new life.

I know that we were not more worthy in any way to be granted the fairy-tale ending that we had. It was just the custom design that was mapped out for us alone. And that is what remains with me until today, the faith that whatever we must experience is directed from Above.

And so it is with gratitude to *Hashem Yisborach* that I am at the point of reading over this manuscript. It surprised me to see the number of references to the times my daughter cried. I reflect back to the time of her illness and I mostly recall her vibrant spirit, her sense of humor, her optimism in all circumstances, and her smile. Particularly ingrained in my mind is how she used to thank me after I injected her with painful shots. When Hashem sends us difficulties He packages them with a measure of strength to counteract them.

Our strength came from witnessing my daughter's acceptance of everything that was decreed upon her. The effects of chemotherapy, her loss of hair, the loss of a social life; each one in and of itself was a cause for depression. My child, however, accepted it all, grew from the adversity, and emerged a mature and self-confident adult.

In reviewing these pages it also struck me that many people involved in our lives during that period were not mentioned in the book. At first we started revising the draft and including those who contributed in any way to making our lives easier at that time. It then occurred to me that this book was about my daughter's viewpoint during her illness. She was really too sick to be concerned about who was learning with her brothers, researching alternative medicine, or arranging for her rides when necessary. And so it was decided to leave the journal as it was written. Besides, if this were to become a book of "thank you's," one book alone would not suffice; we would need volumes. In no way, however, does the lack of mention reflect our lack of appreciation for every single family member, friend, neighbor, stranger, and organization that went out of their way to express concern, give *chizuk*, daven, and help with anything that we needed.

Lastly, I feel that I would be remiss if I did not use this forum to encourage our community to rethink the way they view those who have triumphed over illness, especially when it comes to *shidduchim*. Those who have weathered the storm and come out with a clean bill of health are for the most part as healthy as the average person. I have observed that they usually manifest a maturity beyond their years and a sense of *bitachon* lacking in many "normal" people.

I commend my *mechutanim* for entertaining the *shidduch* with our daughter. They could have easily gone the way of society and rejected a "sick" individual. They consulted with their Rebbe, and subsequently with her doctor, and then gave their blessing. Now the blessing comes their way with *nachas* from our shared grandson. I am confident that we will share much more *nachas* together.

Obviously my thoughts and feelings are well beyond the scope of a foreword. A mother can easily write her own book of what it is like to be along for the ride their child is taking. This is the diary of *my* teenager, who, through her journey in life, blossomed into a most unique individual. I am proud to call her my daughter.

Just a Train of Thought ...

Sometimes I feel like I'm being taken for a ride.
Like in a train.
It follows a set track, built by someone smarter than me
   who knew what he was doing.
Sometimes I have my own ideas about how I'd like my
      train to run, but eventually, you learn that you're not
      the one calling all the stops.
Sometimes the ride is noisy, and sometimes it's o.k.
It just depends on the ground we're covering at that
      point.
Every so often we go through some dark spots.
Sometimes they're frightening, but then we learn that
      they're called tunnels, and that they lead us to places
      we'd never have expected to land up in.
Sometimes I feel like a tunnel is too long and that I'll
      never get out of the dark.

At times like those, we learn to turn around in our seats and focus on the light of the tunnel opening behind us.

And when that eventually fades away into nothing, I can turn around and I can almost always see the light at the end of the tunnel approaching.

Almost always.

And those times when we don't see the light at the end of the tunnel, we just learn to sit back for the dark ride, and we learn to trust the One driving the train.

Because after all, He's the one calling all the stops.

Motza'ei Shabbos, October 25, 2003

Bricks, ASAP, and Augmentin

The first thing that went through my mind was that I must've had a brick in my neck. It was Thursday, at the end of first period, and I was bending down to get my siddur, when suddenly it hurt to move my head.

Instinctively, my hands went to my neck and I felt two big bumps I'd never felt before.

I put down my siddur and felt my neck again and again, all around, and pushed and poked to make sure I wasn't dreaming.

I wasn't.

I turned around to whisper to the girl who sat behind me;

asking her if she saw anything strange about my neck, and she felt my bumps too.

I was reminded of the *Chicken Soup for the Soul* books, where people found bumps and were then diagnosed with cancer. I told that to my friend and we both laughed loud enough for our teacher to hear and ask us to begin davening.

I figured the worst it could possibly be was the result of a tick bite I had gotten over Sukkos vacation.

It wasn't until lunch period that I had a chance to call my parents at work. I waited on line at the pay phone for ages and finally got my turn to call my parents, who weren't too thrilled to hear from me.

We were two sisters in high school at the same time. When Faigy called, it was because she had just gotten some sort of award or the highest score on a test. When I called it was either because I was in trouble or because I wanted to go home.

Okay, I wasn't a troublemaker, but I tried to get out of class a lot. I had had Epstein-Barr virus the year before and I got used to skipping school. I used to call my parents all the time to tell them I felt tired and to try and get permission to go home and miss Chemistry.

Who am I kidding; I was a little monster.

When I told my mother about the bumps, she thought I'd lost my marbles, but I finally convinced her that I knew my own neck and that I really did have a brick inside of it.

My mother wasn't sure if I was faking just to get out of school, so we agreed that if I left school early I would really have to go to the doctor and check it out. I wasn't gaining any free time.

That was fine by me. As long as I got to miss Chemistry, even the doctor was a pleasing alternative.

By the time I left school, even I doubted myself. I had been feeling the bumps all day to make sure they were still there, but by the end of the day, I couldn't tell if they were bumps, or just the way my neck was shaped.

When I told Dr. Rosenberg about my bumps, I think he also thought I was just trying to get out of class. Maybe he was right about the cutting Chemistry part, but when he felt my neck he told me to go to an ear, nose, and throat specialist, "A.S.A.P."

I had to ask him what A.S.A.P. stood for, and he wanted to know how I got to eleventh grade without knowing that.

It turns out it stands for "As Soon As Possible." Who would have guessed? When I asked Faigy if she knew what it stood for, she looked at me in the same way Dr. Rosenberg had and wondered aloud how I ever passed tenth grade.

My little sister and my doctor seemed to have it in for me. Wonderful.

My mother spent the entire night trying to get me an appointment with an ENT (ear, nose, and throat specialist) for Friday. The problem was, we didn't have a referral from Dr. Rosenberg and we couldn't get one until eleven a.m. the next day.

Friday morning I decided that I'd had enough of doctors and referrals and bumps and that I was going to school. I was halfway out the door when my mother found a doctor who had a 1:30 appointment available and a 12:30 appointment, too. She asked me which one I wanted.

I mean, is that even a question? I took the 12:30 and chose to miss school, of course.

It was a good thing I took the 12:30 because we didn't get in to see the doctor until two hours later. Just when I was about to die of either boredom or the smell of the place, I was called into the examining room.

The doctor was a woman who scared me half to death with the expression on her face when she saw my bumps. I thought I was going to die.

Doctors with accents are so much scarier than ones who speak clear English. Everything she said sounded worse because her English was so hard to understand. The doctor prescribed what sounded like a million blood tests and a CT scan, STAT.

I had to ask her what STAT stood for and she said it stood for A.S.A.P. Good thing Dr. Rosenberg had explained that to me the day before!

We couldn't get out of that office soon enough, but as soon as we did, we had to go into the lab next door to do some blood tests.

Big problem. They were closed.

So was the other lab we usually went to, and it was an early Shabbos. We were going nuts.

We called a friend who worked at a local pharmacy, asking him to fill a prescription for Augmentin. The doctor with the accent had said that in case the bumps were the result of some virus, the Augmentin would take care of it. We got the prescription sent over, and then our friend sent us to his friend, another doctor, so that we could hear the diagnosis from a normal person. To me, *normal* meant someone who could tell me what was wrong with me in a language I understood.

Dr. Aaron didn't accept my insurance, but he was nice and only charged us thirty dollars for the visit. He had the coolest books in his basement office; there were tons on history and Jewish philosophy, and also a lot of those "idiot guide" books all over the place.

So I sat on my third examining table in two days, shut my mouth, and let him poke my neck.

The doctor squinted a few times. He peeked over his glasses and then again into his glasses and then he took off his glasses and put them back on before he spoke.

"It's her lymph nodes," he told my mother. I knew what those were. We learned about them in Biology. They were these things in my body that helped me fight infections.

Then the doctor asked if I'd ever had Epstein-Barr virus before. I was amazed at how he knew to ask. I tried looking in the mirror to see if it was stamped on my forehead, but then the doctor told me to be a sweetheart and go wait in the waiting room while he had a talk with my mommy.

Such nerve. I was sixteen. I wasn't a little kid anymore. And for the record: no one gets away with calling me "sweetheart."

My mother didn't tell me what the doctor said, and frankly, I wasn't interested. I was busy thinking about how much work I'd missed in school. I almost flipped when I overheard my mother telling my attendance teacher that I was probably going to miss some more school because I had to go for tests.

I couldn't imagine having to make up so much schoolwork, and play tryouts were scheduled for Sunday. I was *not* going to miss that!

Blood Tests and Play Tryouts

The lab that did my bloodwork was located in a Rite Aid pharmacy that opened at 9 a.m. I was going to have to miss some school, but was hoping to make it back in time for the tryouts.

My mother and I got there at 8:30 Sunday morning just so that we could be the first ones there to sign the waiting list. Because we came so early, we turned out to be the first ones in line after seventeen other people.

I felt bad making my parents come with me all the time and having to wait on all those long lines, but then again, as they never tired of reminding me, at age 16, I was still a minor.

The clerk at the window told us that the technician would arrive shortly. In the meantime I went to explore the Hallmark aisle to look for a birthday card for my father. I was never the kind of girl who liked shopping for funny cards and those kinds of cutesy presents, so after twenty minutes I got bored.

I went back to the lab to see what was going on, but the technician wasn't in yet. I explored for another fifteen minutes, buying cards for my friend Miri, whose birthday wasn't until December, but the tech still hadn't arrived. I think I bought cards for every single girl I ever said "hi" to before I learned that the word "shortly" really meant an hour-and-a-half.

Finally the technician arrived, and she worked very fast. Two hours later my number was called.

I hated being stuck for blood, but this technician took the cake. She was upset at my mother for letting me eat in the morning before the bloodwork and that meant she couldn't concentrate that well on what she was doing. She ended up stabbing me a few times before she got the vein.

I was dizzy for a while, and when the tech asked if I was okay, I had to resist the urge to make a face at her. I know, at sixteen I was very mature. I just yanked my sleeve down and pulled my mother out to the car. I begged her to drive me to school to see if I could still make the play tryouts.

On the way to school, I finally asked my mother about all these tests. She told me that the doctors said that the bumps could be Epstein-Barr-related because EBV has an effect on the lymph nodes. They gave me tests for EBV, mono, CMV, and Lyme disease.

Most people would not test for Lyme, but because I had managed to play host to a deer tick the week before, I had to take that test, just in case. My older sister Chavy was lording that incident over me as if it had only happened because

I hadn't listened to her when she said I was too old to roll down that hill with my siblings when we went apple-picking. My sister acted like she owned me ever since she had gotten married in August.

Chavy and I looked very alike, but we were so different. People used to mix us up all the time, but as soon as I opened my mouth people would know I was anyone but Chavy.

I came to school just in time for the tryouts, but I didn't think I did too well. I was dizzy from giving blood and I was sick from the Augmentin.

Oh yeah, they forgot to tell me that it had side effects.

I took the band-aid off my arm too soon after the blood test just to see how big a black-and-blue mark I could get. I got a nice big one this time, and I paraded it all around school.

Like I said, I was very mature. Most people understood why Chavy and I got along the way we did.

I spent all night making up the work I had missed. Eleventh grade was *so* not a picnic. I had what seemed like twenty-eight teachers and they all piled the homework up as if each was the only instructor we had. I spent a couple of hours talking on the phone, then (out of guilt) a couple of minutes on schoolwork, and then another couple of hours on the phone.

What a day.

CT Scans and the I.C.U

Monday morning I had no doctors to see, so I finally went to school. I can't say I was enjoying myself, but I was doing moderately okay during math, first period, when all of a sudden the door to the classroom burst open.

There stood the secretary. She looked up and down our quiet rows of monsters, students, whatever, then cleared her throat, pointed to me, and read from a small paper.

"Your mother called and said you should not eat anything this morning. I repeat, don't eat anything! Your mother will pick you up in twenty minutes, wait outside for her."

She walked out of the room at the same time that my heart hit the floor. I couldn't decide whether to be mortified at the announcement or to be excited about missing school.

I quickly got over the mortification. I had just been told, "No school for you today, kiddo!" I couldn't have been happier.

Miss Riegler, my Math teacher, asked where I was going. I told her that I had some tests to take care of. She asked me why and I told her because her tests didn't challenge me enough. She was too taken aback to be angry.

Also, I'm too cute for people to get mad at me.

Before taking the CT scan, they make you fast for four hours. I was fine with that, but it turned out that the wait made it more like a six-hour fast for me. There was nothing to read in the waiting room but a bunch of pamphlets about kidney disease, and I couldn't make conversation with the girl next to me because she had her headphones blaring. I was bored and annoyed so I curled up in a plastic chair and took a nap.

When they finally called me in, I had to put on the kind of gown they use in hospitals, the ones they call "I.C.U." because they're open in the back.

There was a huge machine in a brightly lit room that looked kind of like a donut, except it was peach-colored. It was big and round and had a hole in the middle.

I had to lie on a table and not move my head for about fifteen minutes while they scanned my neck.

Then I got jabbed with an IV. The fluid in the IV was iodine. It helped highlight some things in my body so that they showed up clearer on the scan. It made me feel hot all over and my mouth tasted like I was breathing in helium. It was over quickly.

I was driven back to school, where I met the Chumash teacher, who was walking out as I was coming in. She asked where I had gone and I showed her my bumps. She asked me a ton of questions and ended off by telling me that everything was going to be fine and that I shouldn't worry.

I told her that I was not worried in the least. She was shocked. "What do you mean, you're not worried? You have these big bumps on your neck, why aren't you worried?"

And so I ended up spending twenty minutes calming *her* down. Oh, boy!

Tuesday, October 28, 2003

What's a Hematologist?

uesday was just a bad day. I hadn't made up all my work and some teachers were upset with me. When I came home I spent a long time being angry and making up schoolwork (again) until I finally remembered to ask my mother about the results of my CT scan.

I should've asked her sooner because I needn't have bothered with homework. Guess what? No school for me on Wednesday either!

My mother said that the scan showed masses all over my neck and as far down into my chest as the scan showed.

We got in touch with Ezra L'Marpeh, and they set us up with a Dr. Robinson from NYU in Manhattan, He was a hematologist, a doctor who worked with diseases in the blood.

When my mother told me I was going to a hematologist, I was pretty sure that I had cancer. I wasn't really scared of it at that point; it just seemed to be a fact in my mind.

I called my friend Miri and told her everything. She and I didn't go to the same school, so I couldn't keep her updated on every second of my life, even though she's been my best friend since forever.

It was a good thing we were in separate schools; if we had been together the school would have split us up anyway. We looked completely different, but were similar in that we were very grown-up and full of "maturiosity."

Maturiosity is not to be confused with *maturity*. Maturiosity is what we called our own brand of trouble.

Miri was short and petite and had the most angelic face you could imagine on a teenage girl. She had the petite nose and the big eyes and the long eyelashes required for the "I'm perfect" look. Miri used to joke that the closest she came to anything heavenly was that she was a holy terror.

Miri's sister Shaindy was just like my sister Chavy. I always said that Shaindy and Chavy should have gotten to know each other, and then they'd have kept each other so busy talking about our misadventures that they'd forget to bother us.

Miri suggested that we conference-call to Ayala, a camp friend whose younger brother was sick with leukemia. With my best friend on the line, I asked Ayala if her brother's doctor was called a hematologist. She told me what I wanted to know and then asked why I cared.

I told her that a friend of mine was being diagnosed. Ayala, the eternal *tzadekes*, asked me for her name so she could say *Tehillim*. Caught in my lie, I told her that I didn't have the complete name yet, but that I'd give it to her once I had it.

Miri and I spoke until very late that night, discussing the possibility of my having cancer. It was the first conversation we had ever had where we were both close to crying. Miri was sobbing into the phone, saying she couldn't wreak havoc without my help, and I was teary, thinking about not being there to make a mess with her.

We were famous for getting into trouble together. If there was anything exciting going on, you could bet that we were either right there to see it, or were the ones to have caused it.

I was upset about potentially missing out on fun times, but I don't know why I wasn't scared. I was worried, but not terrified. I honestly believed that Hashem knew what He was doing when He sent this test to me. He knew I could handle it, and I didn't doubt for a second He was right. I also didn't think that it was real. Yet.

But I'm jumping ahead of myself.

Wednesday,
October 29, 2003

Elevators
and Bald Heads

*I*t took over an hour to get to Dr. Robinson's office by train, and then some more time to walk to the building.

It took even more time to find out we were in the wrong building, and that meant more time until we found the right one.

How are you supposed to tell those buildings apart? They're all so tall and have so many windows.

As soon as we (finally) walked into the lobby of the right building, we joined a line of about twenty people all waiting for the elevator. Thus began my experience with elevators in

Manhattan. As soon as one arrived, the entire crowd in the lobby rushed into it. That sometimes meant more than thirty people in the tiny crowded box at one time. It got very claustrophobic in there after the doors closed, and that's when they all started reaching over me to push the button for their floor. As the elevator stopped on each floor, more and more people crammed in, using up all the air I was saving for myself.

The whole thing made me kind of nauseated.

Two floors before our stop, we had to start pushing our way out or we'd never make it out in time.

Within two days I became quite the pro at getting people out of my way and getting to my floor on the first try.

My doctor was on the 8th floor in the Oval Center. The elevator opened into a small, cute area, mainly designed for little children. We waited for a long time (standard fare in Manhattan doctor's offices) and I sat and stared at all the kids with bald heads playing on the floor with their IV poles next to them.

I wondered if my mother thought that I would sit there with my eyes shut the whole time. She was a little uncomfortable that I was seeing all the sick children. She still thought I had no idea what was wrong with me. To be honest, to me the bald heads meant they didn't have to blow-dry their hair for school. It seemed like a plus.

I finally got called in just to take my temperature and weigh myself. It made my day to discover that I had grown a full inch and lost four pounds.

Then my day was ruined when I had to take a blood count. The nurse stuck my finger with a sharp thingy and squeezed a lot of blood out to see if I was anemic and a bunch of other things. That part hurt, and in Manhattan, they don't believe in giving out fancy band-aids to teens.

Dr. Robinson was taking care of an emergency (some kid ran home, refusing to take his chemo) so I read a book while we waited. The nurse kept interrupting every five minutes so that I could fill out forms with my entire life story, and to ask me my name. I told my mother that the next time they asked me my name I was going to tell them "Minnie Mouse," but she got so upset just thinking about it that I felt bad and behaved.

After the longest time, I met my doctor. He was the nicest man in the world, and he had once worked together with my pediatrician, Dr. Rosenberg, which I thought was very funny.

My neck got poked again by the doctor and then by his intern. They found another bump under my left arm. After I got dressed again, Dr. Robinson asked me a load of questions like if I was having night sweats, weight loss, fevers, and shortness of breath.

Now that he mentioned it, I *had* been sweating at night. I used to wake up at the oddest hours, drenched. If I'd been sleeping on the bottom bunk I would have gotten up to change, but being on the top bunk meant I was lazy to get down, and most nights I went right back to sleep.

The doctor looked very busy with his papers for a while as I (for a change) waited quietly.

Finally, he told me that he thought I had something called Hodgkin's disease, which was a type of lymphoma, which was a type of cancer.

My mother looked like she was going to burst into tears, and I just sat there with a shocked smile I couldn't wipe off my face. The intern looked at me and said, "He just told you that you have cancer. Why do you look like school was canceled?"

"Because it was!" I beamed.

Just another example of my advanced emotional state. Chavy and Faigy would have denied I was their sister.

I sort of expected it, but hearing it made it real. I was more than a little stunned by the news and I didn't know how to react. I just kept hearing the echo of Dr. Robinson's words running through my head.

He thought I had cancer.

In the next few minutes we found out a lot of things, like who my surgeon should be for a biopsy, what a biopsy was, when it would be done, and why Dr. Robinson's office was full of police officers.

The surgeon was going to be Dr. Ginsberg, the biopsy was a type of surgery, and the police were looking for the boy who ran away from chemo.

Dr. Robinson's secretary, the nicest woman in the world, got us an immediate appointment with the surgeon, Dr. Ginsberg.

We had to go back into the elevator, out of the building, up the block, around the corner, across the street, halfway down another block, into the hospital, make a right to the elevator, go up to the tenth floor, fill out forms, and take a seat for an hour.

I read two magazines before I met the other nicest man in the world, Dr. Ginsberg. He also felt my bumps (which were pretty sore by then) and told me about my biopsy.

It would take place in two days, on Friday, at 10:15 a.m., on the tenth floor on the other side of the building and I would be an outpatient, which meant I could go home right after the surgery.

They were going to make a small cut on my neck, about an inch long, and then they were going to cut out a little bit of one of my bumps to test it to see if it was really Hodgkin's. After that, they would stitch me back up, and that was it.

It didn't sound too bad.

Chavy was over at our house trying to get everyone in order when we got home. She was upset at Faigy because she was obsessing over her homework instead of helping out with the kids. When I walked through the door she was annoyed at me for being the cause of my mother's absence. She was not even twenty yet and she thought she owned the rights to my life.

My mother told her quietly what the doctor told us and Chavy's whole attitude changed. Yay. Cancer made me worth being nice to. About time she realized I was special!

I called Miri to tell her what the doctor said, and then I called Devoiry and Suri and Meira. I spent most of the night comforting them and promising I wasn't going to die and I was so busy comforting them, I didn't have time to think about comforting myself.

Life can be so ironic.

Thursday, October 30, 2003

My Happy Hodgkin's Day

I had been looking forward to Thursday ever since I was in ninth grade. It was the day of our big sister–little sister skating trip and I was finally on the "big sister" side of things.

The big sister–little sister partners were a G.O.-organized event. The idea was to pair each freshman and sophomore in the school with someone in either the junior or senior classes. The big sisters were there to help the little ones make any adjustments that they found difficult in high school.

Once a year we took a trip to the roller-skating rink so that the "sisters" could pair up and skate together and get to know each other while zooming and falling over everyone else.

I was having a great time until we got off the bus. After five minutes on the rink, some Freshie knocked into me and caused me to fall, twisting my neck.

My neck had been sore to begin with, but now I was really in pain. I spent the rest of the day sitting on the bench at the side, watching everyone else skate.

I had a big headache and it got bigger every time someone else asked me to skate with her. Eventually, I just let my friend borrow my blades and put my shoes back on.

My day got worse when my neighbor Meira started to talk to me about my hair falling out. I had known that I would be bald, but Meira pointed out that I would lose my eyebrows too. I didn't think they made wigs for that. I was depressed the entire way home.

I didn't want to eat supper, and when my mother asked me why, I started crying, and so did she. She took me down to an empty room in the basement where we could talk, and that extra attention made my brothers insanely jealous.

I cried for a long time, and I felt better when I was finished. I asked my mother if the chemotherapy I would take would affect my health in the future. My mother said she didn't know what to tell me, and then we cried for another half-hour.

All my friends who knew what was going on called to see how I was doing and to get some more reassurance from me that everything was going to be fine. I told them that everything was going to be okay, and then my parents went online to find out more about what I had.

They found some really great websites that explained things very well.

There was this one site, "Dave's Happy Hodgkin's Website," that kept us laughing all night. A boy about my age who had gone through Hodgkin's described his experience very well, in a reader-friendly and even funny way.

Of course, we didn't understand many of the things we read until we actually went through them later, but the information we found and the humorous tone made us all feel better that night.

We learned that Hodgkin's was probably the most curable form of cancer. It's found only in the lymph nodes in the beginning, but then it may spread. Because it isn't found in any major organs, the chance of lasting damage is very slim.

Twenty years ago, this disease was treated with a huge dose of radiation and chemo, thereby increasing the risk of infertility and other cancers later in life. But today, after years of research, they have been able to cut down on the radiation and chemo, and the risks are much smaller.

It didn't change the fact that I would lose a lot of weight and my hair. That is pretty traumatic for anyone to go through, but more so for a sixteen-year-old girl. I told everyone that I didn't care, and that I wanted to wear a hat all the way down over my face instead of getting a sheitel, but I really did care.

I was a JAP. I was the girl who loved everything about being a girl. The clothing, the shoes, the makeup, the shoes, the accessories, the shoes, the jewelry, the shoes, doing my long dark hair, the shoes, and did I mention the shoes? My days as a JAP seemed to be changing into my days as a JACP. A Jewish American Princess turning into a Jewish American Cancer Patient.

I cared a lot.

Friday, October 31, 2003

Biopsy: A Literal Pain in the Neck

We took a cab to NYU the next morning, took the "A" elevator up to the day-surgery ward, filled out a zillion forms with my autobiography, waited, read books, waited some more, and cried.

I don't know why, but as I was reading, something made me start thinking of what it meant to really have cancer, and then I remembered all my questions from the night before, and I just began to bawl — right there in the waiting room.

A bunch of people were staring at me and a few looked sorry. My mother also started to cry a little, so I stopped crying to make her stop too.

I got a hospital bracelet, had enough time to memorize my ID number (0169120), and then I was called into the surgery prep.

My mother came with me into a teensy weensy little room and then waited in the hallway while I got undressed and put on two hospital gowns, the first open in the back, and the second open in the front. I had to put on a shower cap kind of thing that felt like the strips of Bounce we used in the dryer. I also got the Bounce things in booties for my feet. They were disgusting, but sneakers weren't allowed on the operating table.

My regular clothing was put into a private locker and then a group of nurses came to speak to me. Of course, they all had to take turns coming in, because the cubicle I was in was so small. Because they weren't all in there at the same time, they all ended up asking the same questions over and over again.

If I thought I looked silly in my new hospital garb, the nurses all looked worse. They were all dressed in blue scrub suits, really ugly, with bunchy waistbands and big pockets. The hairnet I had to wear was part of their uniform too, but they didn't wear booties. They wore some kind of weird white slippers that looked like plastic clogs.

I hadn't been allowed to eat from midnight the night before, and that was a good thing. I was so nervous; I would've thrown up anything I'd eaten anyway, all over my beautiful gown. The reason they don't let patients eat before surgery is because when a person is under anesthesia, the entire body stops working. They want to make sure that no food is stuck down there when the machinery shuts down.

That can be dangerous.

My sense of humor returned once I started meeting the doctors. Again, they kept asking me my name every couple of minutes, and again I was tempted to say "Mother Goose," but my mother had given me a strict warning beforehand.

That didn't stop me from acting crazy, though. When the anesthesiologist, a really nice person, Max or Mark or Matt or whatever, asked me what I was allergic to, I told him, "School."

I met about three nurses, the anesthesiologist, Dr. Ginsberg the surgeon, and some other people who all had us fill out forms and sign our consent for the operation.

One nurse asked if I ate normally. My mother told her I ate like a teenager, so that's what the nurse wrote on the form.

The staff told us a whole bunch of do's and don'ts about surgery. Mostly *don'ts*, like don't eat, don't wear jewelry, and don't wear contact lenses during surgery.

When I got into the operating room, the nurses welcomed me and called me "Honey" and "Sweetheart." I carefully checked my hospital bracelet and told the nurse that I must be in the wrong room because that wasn't the name I had on my wrist. They thought I was funny, but I said it in all seriousness. No one gets away with calling me "Honey."

When we got my identity crisis all figured out, the nurses had me lie down on the operating table. Dr. Ginsberg made a couple of X's on my neck so that he'd remember where to cut. I found it very frightening that the doctor thought he had to make lines so that he'd remember where my bumps were when we had already discussed it and when he already had a chart with a diagram hanging above my bed.

He joked that he needed lines to show him how to cut straight because he had been a horror with the scissors in kindergarten.

I found that even more upsetting.

Then they knocked me out.

My surgeon and my anesthesiologist had discussed this with me before. I was hit with general anesthesia, which puts the whole body out, as opposed to local anesthesia, which only numbs certain parts of the body. I had a choice of an IV or a gas mask, and of course, I chose the mask.

It was so cool. I was out like a light.

I woke up as soon as the surgery was over. I didn't believe that they had even started on me, so I tried to get off the table. The pain in my neck made me lie right back down.

I was in a lot of pain, and really nauseated. My mother was all worried because I was feeling so sick. It turned out that they had forgotten to open my IV line all the way and I wasn't getting enough fluid. After an hour-and-a-half, they gave me meds to ease the pain, and after almost an hour of meds and a mandatory trip to the bathroom, I was free to go.

It was hard to get dressed because of my stitches, but I did it myself. I managed to eat some gross saltines because my mother made me, and I even made it to the elevator alone.

As soon as the elevator doors closed, we had a problem. I blacked out from the nausea and the pain. The people in the elevator got me down to the lobby, where they put me into an armchair, and my mother found us a ride back home with a *chesed* organization.

I don't remember much about the day. They warned me at the hospital that I would experience some minor discomfort. I learned then that "minor discomfort" really meant dire pain for three days.

At the hospital they kept asking me to rate my pain on a scale of one to ten. I was brave and kept telling them that I felt like a two, but they only brought me a painkiller when I told them eight, just to see what they would do.

I was asked this question every forty-five seconds.

Well, as soon as I came home I felt like a ten, so I went up to bed. Or at least I tried to, because all the people who knew I was having a biopsy called me.

I got so many calls, I cried every time the phone rang. I

know everyone just meant well, but it got very tiring for me and for my family.

The one call I did appreciate was a call from a random classmate who had no idea that anything was wrong. Raizy Freund was just being nice and called to see why I was absent. It touched me that she didn't want anything more from me than just that.

Just as a side note, in the two weeks since this story began, not a single girl in my entire class had bothered to notice that I was gone every other day. No one had called and even when I was back in school, no one asked me where I had been.

As a teenager myself I understood them. I didn't expect to be called by anyone who wasn't in my immediate circle of friends. That's the way it works in high school. I had lots of friends. I knew I was popular, I always was. It's just that most girls don't think of calling when someone else is absent. Most of the time, no one notices when a girl is out for a day or two.

But when Raizy called, it made me stop and think.

Raizy was the type of girl everyone in school wanted to be. She was head of the school choir, and she ran for the G.O. the year before and she was just one of the girls who made the whole high-school experience so enjoyable. She was part of the group who planned all our fun and was so popular that if she hadn't been so nice people would have been afraid to be her friend.

But that was it. Maybe part of her popularity was due to the fact that she was nice. She was busy but still took the time to notice when a classmate was out for a few days and then made it her business to call.

When I was sending out my wedding invitations way after this story was over, I didn't invite classmates I had lost touch with. I had nothing to do with Raizy Freund either, but I sent her an invitation anyway. In her invite, I wrote to her about what an impression she had made on me by calling that Friday. Some classmates thought I was a snob for not inviting each one of them personally, but they really couldn't understand what it felt like to have been a sixteen-year-old girl who came out of surgery one Friday thinking that as popular as she was, no one really cared about her.

Anyway, that's jumping ahead of myself. Getting back to Friday, I couldn't even take a shower for Shabbos because my stitches were still raw. Tired and smelly, and still in a lot of pain, I made it to *licht bentchen.*

Friday night, I was taking care of my "minor discomfort" by sleeping on the couch, when my neighbors knocked on my door.

Big problem. I had forgotten that I had promised to babysit for them that night while they went to their daughter's Shabbos *sheva berachos.* They had booked me a week in advance, but it had totally slipped my mind with everything else that was going on.

As far as I was concerned, a week ago could have been last millennium. My life had changed so much since then.

My sister Faigy had a big test to study for and my brother Zevy was too young to babysit so late, so I ran around the neighborhood looking for a replacement, but to my mazal, I ended up having to leave in the middle of my meal to babysit till about 11 p.m.

Thankfully, my neighbor Meira came along to help and keep me company and that made the time pass quicker.

That week was a literal pain in the neck.

Monday,
November 03, 2003

Diagnosis and Some Creepy Coincidences

onday was so weird.

As soon as Morah Templer saw me walk into the school, she ran over to me and gave me a big hug and a kiss in front of everyone in the *entire* hallway. That is probably the biggest violation of teenager-hood, if there ever was one. It is the cardinal no-no to let oneself be hugged — and be hugged in *public* — and by a *teacher* no less.

During lunch, I was called over by the *mechaneches* of the grade for a "get to know you" meeting and she asked a bunch of personal questions. She had heard about me from some other teachers who said I was having a little bit of an attitude problem.

Take the first day of school for example:

There was one teacher who was famous for her "first day of school lesson." She did the same thing every year. She would walk into a classroom, point to one girl, and say, "YOU!!!" That year she made the mistake of pointing at me.

"You," she said, "do you love G-d?"

I looked at her and answered, "No, I don't think so."

I didn't mean that I didn't have *ahavas Hashem*. I meant that I knew I wasn't up to the level of *ahavas Hashem* that she was trying to bring out. I knew that she expected me to say that I loved Hashem, and then she was going to disprove it by telling me that a sixteen-year-old couldn't possibly reach perfection in that area. It was what she did every year. I wasn't going to give her the satisfaction of making me feel stupid on the first day of class. So I was honest with her.

The teacher was taken aback by my answer. "Let me ask you this then, do you follow His commandments?"

"Sure."

The teacher's face lit up as if she had just invented the light bulb. "If you don't love G-d, then why do you do His mitzvos?"

"Well, I do your homework," I answered.

The class was roaring. I was kicked out.

Yeah, well, I guess I did have an attitude problem ....

I think the *mechaneches* was very interested in me, and I played up that meeting to the fullest. She asked me a load of questions, and I just wouldn't give her serious answers. She was so shocked later when she found out that I was sick. She thought I was way too hyper to take anything in life seriously.

Maybe she just happened to be right.

I still had time after that to joke around with some friends, forget to eat, and get a note telling me to call my mother. I asked the secretary if I could use the office phone and she said, "No. Who do you think you are?" So I went downstairs to the basement and waited on a long line to use the payphone near the janitor's office. Closet. Whatever.

By the time I got the phone, the bell for the next period was ringing, so I was rushing not to be late to class. Finally, I got past three secretaries, a voicemail, and two extensions, and my mother got on the line and then handed me over to my father because she had another call.

My father told me that based on what came up in the preliminary results of my biopsy, they weren't even going to do any further testing. I had Hodgkin's.

I didn't even bother running up the three flights of stairs to computer class, because I was already late, and I didn't think that in my current mood, coming another minute late would matter. So I dragged myself upstairs, let myself get yelled at, and then started doing the class assignment.

In the middle of the lesson, the girl who sat near me turned around to ask me whatever had happened to those bumps on my neck that I had shown her in class around two weeks before.

I was in no mood to be yelled at again, so without looking away from the computer screen, I whispered to her that I had cancer. The girl let out a shriek that was heard all the way down the stairs. The entire class looked at her and she just shrieked again.

When the teacher demanded to know what was wrong, I just told her that we had both made it to callbacks for the play, and were very excited.

My friend got a demerit, and the privilege of having my life remain private was extended until the end of the class.

It was true that I had made it to callbacks, but it didn't even feel as good as I expected it to. I was finally getting my chance to get on stage and do what I loved, but I knew that whether I got the lead role or just one sentence, I wouldn't make it to the play anyway. It hurt.

During recess, I heard a huge commotion coming from my classroom, and I really wasn't interested to know why. My maturiosity told me that I had enough of my own problems to deal with and that I didn't have to go and listen to a bunch of girls shriek about a test or something equally stupid.

Turns out they were all shrieking about *me*. The girl sitting next to me during computers had gone and told everyone that I had a brain tumor, for heaven's sake. I quickly said that I had something way different, and that it was no big deal.

One girl piped up and said, "But we heard you had, you know, '*yene machlah*'!"

"And so?"

"So it's true?"

I just looked at her and said, "Well, yeah."

The class started shrieking again.

So now it wasn't enough that I had an unspeakable illness, I also had to go deaf.

After school I went over to my math teacher, Miss Riegler, to ask her for the best book to use to keep up with the Regents curriculum if I had to be out of school for a while.

She thought I was taking a holiday in Florida or something, so she was smiling when she gave me the name of a book she recommended. She asked me how long I planned to be gone, and when I told her about four to five months, she just cracked up. She thought I was joking.

All of a sudden, the entire class knew my telephone number. That night, about forty people called for me. Now that I had cancer, I was worth the call. I was a celebrity now, not just some anonymous classmate who had missed a few days of school.

That made me a little upset. These girls hadn't cared to call me at home before they heard I had cancer, and now they all wanted to be my best friend. I felt that people were gravitating toward me because the closer they got to me, the closer they were going to get to the center of attention.

I know it isn't fair to say so of girls who only meant well. But I was hurt that all the well-meaning people showed up only after they heard I was ill. If they really meant well for me, where were they when I was just another face in the crowd? Or was I just not worth knowing then?

Okay, I wasn't just another face in the crowd. I was always popular and in the center of things, but sometimes the popular girls only have a few close friends. Everyone always knew my name and I never had any problems making new friends and fitting in wherever I went, but as friendly and as "out there" as I was, there were only a few girls to whom I was really close.

It was nice to see how many people wanted to talk to me that night, but it didn't feel right that it had happened all of a sudden. I felt that now my privacy had been taken away from me and that my life wasn't just between me and my friends anymore, it was out there for anyone who wanted to talk about it and make decisions about it and say, "*Oy, nebech.*"

All the cousins found out that night too. All of a sudden I went from being a little cousin to a big celebrity; from a little monster to a bigshot.

We also heard that a lot of rumors started spreading that night. Everyone heard the news from someone who wasn't supposed to know, who heard it from someone who wasn't supposed to tell, who heard it from someone else. I got calls that night from people I hadn't heard from in years. They all called because they heard I had a brain tumor ....

My real friends found it really hard to deal with. People kept coming over to them and asking stupid questions. My friends were pretty annoyed about the constant badgering, but they used it to my advantage when they asked every person who came over to them to join a group of girls who were saying *Perek Shirah* for my recovery.

As the *choleh*, I said I would supply some of the *Perek Shirah* booklets. I mentioned this to my neighbor, Ruchy Perlstein, whose grandfather owned a small Judaica store close to where I lived. Twenty minutes later, she called me to tell me that I was entitled to a free shopping spree in the store. I was thrilled!

Here's where things started getting interesting.

My father's mother, the grandmother I was named after, had her *yahrtzeit* on the coming Tuesday. Not sure if he'd make it to the cemetery then, my father went up on Sunday. While he was there, he noticed that one of the letters in my grandmother's name on her tombstone wasn't whole. The *aleph* in her name had not been chiseled out properly.

My father took a picture of it and sent it to a Rav together with my name. He wanted to ask the Rav what to do about the *matzeivah* and also ask for a *berachah* for me. Right away, the Rav said that an incomplete *aleph* is not such a small deal.

An *aleph* is a very whole letter. It's made up of two *yuds* and a *vav*. The numeric value of these letters is twenty-six, the same as Hashem's name — *Yud- Hey- Vav- Hey*.

What happened on the tombstone was that the "top *yud*" was not connected to the rest of the letter. 26 - 10 = 16 ... my age.

I don't understand much about this kind of stuff, but it was still spooky.

My grandmother died when she was very young, when my father was just nine years old, and even though everyone named for her had been given an added name as an extra *zechus*, it was a little scary to think of what goes into a name. All the cousins named after this grandmother were having a bad year. One cousin was *niftar*, another was having a very hard pregnancy, and now I was ill.

Later that night, a perfect stranger called my father to ask him if he was going to the cemetery on Tuesday morning, because he wanted to form a *minyan* so he could say *Kaddish* at his parent's grave. He said that he'd help my father make a *minyan* at my grandmother's grave if my father joined the *minyan* for his parent.

It occurred to my father that even though he couldn't make it to the cemetery Tuesday morning because of an appointment with me, he could arrange a *minyan* to be there in the afternoon. While it was still on his mind, he mentioned it to our Rav, and our Rav said that he should surely go out to the cemetery with a group to say *Kaddish,* because it was a really good thing to be there on the day of a *yahrtzeit.*

In the 35 years since my grandmother died, there had never been a *minyan* there at her *kever* on her *yahrtzeit* to say *Kaddish.*

Wanting to find out more about his mother, my father started to call up his mother's sister, but then decided not to tell her anything and make her worry for nothing. He also didn't want her to know that I was sick. He didn't know how she would handle it.

My great-aunt called him a half-hour later. She had had a feeling that something was wrong.

My friend Miri also had her share of coincidences that night. In a small depression about my situation, she tried to distract herself by cleaning her room. When she was going through her CD collection she found an unlabeled disc and put it into the boom box. It turned out to be a *shiur* on what to do when your friend is sick in the hospital. She called me up crying.

Anyway, I was in a rush to get to the bookstore before the Perlsteins changed their mind about my shopping spree, so I told Miri that she could have me in mind until I could find the time for a good cry. Then I shut the phones and dragged my mother out.

I picked up some *Perek Shirah* booklets and a CD while my mother explored.

If we hadn't been getting this stuff for free, this never would have happened. My mother picked up a copy of *Guard Your Tongue,* even though we already had a copy at home. She figured that our copy was a hundred years old and Faigy needed to use it every night for school, so she might as well get another one.

I noticed a lady watching us, and then she finally tapped my mother on her shoulder.

"That book is a book of *refuos* and *yeshuos.* If you learn two *halachos* a day, the Manchester Rosh Yeshivah promised *yeshuos.* I've used it too."

My mother was slightly shocked and asked what the lady had used it for.

"A few years ago my husband was diagnosed with Hodgkin's." I think my jaw still hurts from hitting the floor.

It turned out that this lady never even shopped in this store, she always went to the bigger Jewish bookstore that was near all the shops, but just today her bus had dropped her off in the wrong place and she was exploring the bookshelves until her son came to pick her up.

Coincidences? Or just Hashem showing me He was there all the time?

Tuesday, November 04, 2003

Port-o-What?

uesday was a very busy day. I had another CAT scheduled for 12:00, so I wasn't allowed to eat anything since the morning. The CAT this time was supposed to be more detailed than the last one. My first CAT scan only showed my neck, but this one was going to show all the masses inside of me, down through my entire body. The doctors wanted to see how far down the cancer had spread.

Both my parents came to Dr. Robinson with me so that my father could meet him and so that we could outline my schedule for the rest of the week. Then my father went back to the cemetery for his mother's *yahrtzeit*. He took along his own *minyan* of his brothers and some family to daven there.

My mother and I went on to meet my surgeon for yet another surgery. Dr. Ginsberg, my original surgeon, was away for the week, so we went to meet Dr. Massre.

Dr. Massre was the youngest doctor I had ever met. His hair was still black, and he didn't wear glasses!

He sat with me and explained everything about my surgery. It was called a bone-marrow biopsy, and it was a test to see if the cancer had spread to my bones. He showed me the needle he was going to use to get marrow out of me and it was cool in a gory sort of way. It looked like an apple corer; a long stick with a metal circle at the end of it. I tried to picture him scooping out marrow from my bones with that, but I stopped when I made myself dizzy.

He was going to take the marrow from my lower back and the doctor said that it might cause some minor discomfort.

"Does that really mean that I won't be able to sit for a week?" I asked.

"Boy, you catch on quick!" He laughed and said I could get some painkillers if I needed them.

Another part of my surgery would be to install a metaport, or what's sometimes called a "port-o-cath," into my chest.

Dr. Massre showed me one. It looked like a small half-metal, half-plastic, white stethoscope. It was small and round with a long thin tube attached. The tube went into a vein and the round part got put into a hollow in my chest, right under my shoulder.

Usually, the port is put into the center of the chest, right under the collarbone, but because I was a teen and Dr. Massre was worried about how the scarring would look when I wore a low-cut dress, he was going to put it on the side where I could always cover the scar with the straps of the dress. He told me that I could never wear something strapless because of the scars.

I told him that I didn't think that would ever be a problem for me, and then we had to get into a whole discussion about the laws of *tzniyus* and why I would never wear something low-cut or strapless anyway. He was amazed that we really dressed that way all the time. He didn't even know that they made gowns that had shoulders and sleeves and kosher necklines!

The port was going to be used for chemotherapy. Instead of having to thread an IV line into my hand or arm every time I went for chemo, they could just poke the needle into my chest. It sounded terrible, but supposedly it was less painful that way.

We were just leaving his office when we got a call to run back to Dr. Robinson's place. They had forgotten to take blood from me, and since my CT was pushed off to 2:00 p.m. they figured I could just hop on over.

After waiting for an hour, a nurse in training took six tubes of blood from my poor right arm, which was by then barely recognizable due to the many puncture marks I already had.

I fainted after the fourth tube, so they gave me a break, and then a regular nurse took the other two tubes of blood from me. I was hurting and I was weak, but I couldn't even eat anything because of my upcoming CT scan.

The nurses left the IV line in me because the CT place needed to stick me too, so instead of the pain of another stick, they only made me suffer the discomfort of a needle in my arm for the next six hours.

Yeah, the next six hours.

My mother and I ran like crazy to make it in time to my scan, but by then we should have learned that it wasn't worth it. They didn't even sneeze in our direction till about 3:00 p.m.

From 3:00-4:00 I had to drink a cup of something that tasted like melted taffy. It was totally disgusting. At 4:30, they took me into the scan room.

The CT was the same procedure as last time. I had to wear a hospital gown and take off everything metal and lie very still on the table while it slid me into the donut machine to scan my body.

I got the iodine again, and it made me feel hot and weird, and then they made me drink a liquid that was at least 100 times gassier than seltzer. The gas in it was supposed to make my stomach appear bigger on the scan. They warned me not to burp because then my stomach would shrink again. Whoever invented that stuff obviously never tried that himself. It was pure torture to keep from letting out all those gas bubbles for twenty minutes.

On the way out of the hospital we passed the gift shop, and something in the window caught my eye. It was a pen that had a Bop-It game on top of it. My sister Faigy was obsessed with Bop-It and I thought it was a cute present to thank her for babysitting. My mother liked it too, so we bought it for her.

We took the train back home, and didn't get there till about 7:30 p.m. I felt faint because I hadn't eaten all day and from having all that blood taken.

Of course, there were no seats on the train because of rush hour, and I had to faint again in order to get one.

My sister Chavy was babysitting again and she was starting to hate me for infringing on her *shanah rishonah*. I couldn't understand why Faigy couldn't help out more; she was, after all, in tenth grade already, but Faigy then started going at me, saying that she had a life too and that I was a selfish brat for getting sick and causing them all to suffer.

Ouch.

As soon as I came home I had to field a hundred phone calls. I spoke to Morah Templer and I asked her to please tell everyone to stop calling me and to send me letters instead. I finally took the phone off the hook and ate my first meal of the day at 8:00 p.m.

I didn't mind it when my friends called. Problem was; it wasn't my friends who were calling. My real friends understood that I was tired and didn't want to talk to anyone. The people who called were my "new best friends" who wanted to speak to me because I was now famous.

I had a ton of people calling all at once. It was like they all had to get their fifteen minutes of fame in by being able to say that they had spoken to me the other night.

I considered hiring a public-relations firm to field all my calls. I would have started looking for a PR company but instead of getting a dial tone when I picked up the handset, all I got were some more incoming calls.

Wednesday, November 05, 2003

Surgery Again

We took a cab early in the morning to NYU for surgery. Faigy wasn't too happy about babysitting at 6:00 a.m., but she didn't really have a choice.

Once we got to the hospital, I again had to put on the gown and the shower cap and booties. I met a million people again who all wanted my name, address, telephone number, and the last time I got kicked out of class.

I was so tired; I must've answered "Donald Duck" to at least one person on the team. They themselves were so tired, they probably didn't even notice.

I was looking forward to this operation so that I could lie down on that table and just sleep. No nerves this time.

In the operating room they glued on EKG (electrocardiogram) stickers that would monitor my heart rate throughout my surgery. Those stickers left black-and-blue marks on me for about a week after the procedure.

I got stuck with an IV line and then suddenly the surgery was over.

This time I felt great! Except for some "minor discomfort" in my chest area, I was okay. I got asked the same, "on a scale of one to ten how are you feeling," question every three seconds, and my answer every time was a two.

They warned me about minor discomfort, and this time I knew to ask for a prescription of Tylenol with codeine.

Everything was going great as I was getting dressed, until I looked down and saw a huge piece of Tegaderm (waterproof hospital tape) covering a bloody bandage right under my left shoulder blade. I felt faint and had to sit down to finish buttoning my shirt.

My shirt, by the way, had become a joke in the hospital. I was known as the kid who always wore blue shirts. I had about ten blue shirts that I had worn as a uniform in elementary school and they were soft and easy to put on and take off, so I lived in them during the year I was sick.

Today I never wear light blue. It makes me think of chemotherapy.

I don't remember much after I got dressed, but I was told that I blacked out in the elevator again and then someone drove us to my parents' office building, where I found a couch and slept for about four hours.

On the way home, my mother bought me a huge milkshake, but I couldn't drink it because I felt so sick.

To go-off topic again: I still cannot drink milkshakes to this day. Every time I try to taste one, I taste the chemo in my mouth and I feel the nausea I felt during those times, all over again.

I try to tell patients on chemo to avoid their favorite foods while they are being treated, because when they get better, they will never be able to look at those foods again.

After the milkshake, my neighbor Mrs. Lander took me to get a sheitel made. I was so tired and nauseous that I begged her to just forget it and do it another night, but we went anyway.

I was so depressed sitting in that chair, trying on sheitel after sheitel, trying to get something that matched my hair color exactly, and all the while picturing myself bald.

When the *sheitelmacher* suggested going with a wig a shade lighter than my hair and with some blonde highlights, I'd had enough. I gave up on the whole sheitel idea and said I'd rather go around bald than wear something that didn't look like it was mine.

I had hair that was a unique shade of dark brown. It had the most stunning red highlights that I was so proud of, and I had been growing my hair long over the past year, so it was long, curly, and it was all mine. I could never imagine giving it up for a different color or style.

I convinced Mrs. Lander to just take me home and we would pursue the sheitel thing another night.

I was dying to get to bed, but it didn't seem like an option once I got home. Again I had to deal with a ton of phone calls.

One of the calls I picked up that night was from Etty Gruen. She had gone through chemo for a tumor a few years back. She answered a ton of questions for me and warned me not to eat foods I liked and all the little things I needed to know about chemo.

I ignored all the other calls I had that night, and after talking with Etty, I just went to bed.

Motza'ei Shabbos, November 08, 2003

My Big Fat Week of Scans

ompared to Wednesday, Thursday's bone scan was a breeze.

We waited forty-five minutes until the technician on duty gave me an injection, and then we had to wait three hours for the shot to travel through my system so that we could take the scan. My mother and I found the Bikur Cholim room where my mom took a nap and I was bored for three hours.

Finally, we went back to take the scan, and I was told to lie down on a teensy little table and not to move.

When I heard the test would take a full forty-five minutes, I asked them to strap me to the table because I knew I could not keep still for that long. So they strapped me down and then a bunch of panels began moving around me very slowly. They were scanning my bones to see if the cancer had affected them in any way. It was kind of boring not being able to move or talk, so I just went to sleep.

Friday, we went to Manhattan again and waited in a small waiting room with a family of Chinese people who had accompanied their grandmother to her scan. It seems that family was very close because the entire extended family (there must have been about twenty-five people there) came to take the grandma to her PT scan.

It took less than two minutes for my mother and me to go crazy from the way they were speaking. Their chatter, unintelligible to me, was really getting on my nerves. I was so relieved when I was called in.

The scan itself was similar to the CT scan. This scan was a little more advanced, and it showed the same infections the CT scan showed, but they showed more detail and were able to tell if the masses were tumorous.

The opening in the machine was smaller than the one for the CT, and it was a little claustrophobic to get in there at first. But after my head was done being scanned and it was out of the machine, I felt a little better.

The machine was in a trailer parked on the street because their building was undergoing construction and they had no place to put the machine for the time.

As I was being scanned, I heard the cars and trucks and the city traffic outside. It was cool, but kind of weird to imagine that I was getting a scan done right in the middle of the street.

I liked this scan more than the CT because I didn't need to wear a gown and I was allowed to wear metal.

While the technician helped me put my hands above my head (I couldn't do it myself because my surgery site was still hurting me) she asked me if I had any siblings. I told her that I was the second of ten and she almost dropped my IV line.

During the scan, the technician and I spoke about what it was like to grow up in a family with so many kids. She kept saying that I was so normal; she never would have imagined me from a large family.

I'm left wondering … is something supposed to be wrong with me? Is every kid from a large family supposed to be ab-normal?

When I finally got home, I had to deal with a lot of people who wanted to come and visit me over Shabbos. I kept telling them that I was way too tired for visitors, but they all insisted on coming.

I finally lost my cool and told them if they were coming for me, they weren't doing any mitzvos because I really did not want visitors. If they were coming to alleviate their guilty con-sciences, they were welcome to walk out all the way to my house and I was going to sleep while they cried at my front door.

They got the message, but it took them a half-hour and left me peeved. I know I wasn't very nice about it; they only wanted to be good to me, but with all the *chesed* that they wanted to do, they didn't ever stop to think about how I was really feeling. I was too sick to be up to entertaining visitors, and I don't think they understood that.

My father's sister Carla still hadn't known that I was sick, but my father told her that day because she had called him with the strangest dream. She had dreamed that she saw her late father, my grandfather, smiling and nodding at her, in the best of health. He seemed very happy about something and was dressed very well, as if he were on the way to a wedding.

He didn't speak at all in the dream, but kept smiling broadly and nodding.

She told it to my father, who decided it was because he had gone out to the cemetery and fixed his mother's *matzeivah* — the *matzeivah* that my grandfather had ordered for her.

She had that dream the exact night of my grandmother's *yahrtzeit*: the tenth of Cheshvan.

I don't know what to believe, but it makes a nice story, so I put it down here.

The creepiest part is that my cousin, whose name is also Carla, had a similar dream that same night. She saw both her father and my grandfather dressed up and smiling and proud.

I have a funny family.

That night, after the Shabbos meal, my father's friend Mendy Berger came over with his daughter, who was now in remission for Hodgkin's. He wanted us to see a live sample of what I could look like after I was all better. Nechy was adorable, and she had a head full of curly hair that was as soft as baby hair. She said that after her hair grew back, it felt brand-new, like a baby's.

She answered a lot of my questions, but then I asked her if she had any pictures of when she was sick. She looked at her parents and then the father said to me, "We don't have any pictures of that time. Those are six months we erased from her life."

I was so bothered by that comment that it stayed in my mind for days afterward.

I felt that Hashem knew what he was doing when he made me, of all people sick, and that He was trying to teach me something. Who was I to just "erase from my life" the message I was being sent?

Besides — this was my life! How could I just erase this time and pretend it never happened? What would the world look like if divorced people just "forgot" they were divorced? Would it make getting remarried easier? How about if terminally ill people "forgot" that they were sick? Would it stop them from dying?

I decided that I was not going to forget this time in my life. Ever.

From then on I carried a camera wherever I went. I took pictures of everything. I snapped pictures of surgeries and of the chemo and of my bald head. I even had my mother take a picture of me when I fainted in the emergency room once!

My mother and I created a beautiful scrapbook of all the pictures we had taken while I was sick and now I go around and show it to newbies who are just starting treatment. It makes such a difference to these kids to be able to actually see what they'll be going through. I smiled for every picture, so the scrapbook is more funny than scary, and I still like to look back at it every once in a while just to make sure that I'll never forget what it was like to be a sixteen-year-old with cancer.

Motzaei Shabbos, Chavy took me and Faigy to the mall and I happened to bump into some girls I knew from school. They all looked at me as if I were a ghost. I made some faces and watched them turn blue. I was depressed the rest of the time.

I had a big talk with my mother that night.

She couldn't decide whether to switch to a Dr. Michael Harris in New Jersey, and I couldn't decide if I should scream or cry or both. This doctor was recommended by many people, but my mother didn't want to leave Dr. Robinson.

I really felt I needed to scream, but I didn't want to wake the house up.

My mother was a little upset that this doctor didn't accept new patients very often.

I was upset because a girl I didn't get along with was given a major part in the school play while I didn't get to be in it at all.

My parents couldn't make a decision, and I was mad because everyone was making decisions for me.

I told my parents to try and get me an appointment at this new doctor, and my father told me to try not to open the front door anymore because otherwise I could catch a cold now that my immune system was weak.

After a lot of indecision on my parent's part, and after a lot of venting by me, we all decided to go to sleep. We were all feeling much better.

Amazing what communication can accomplish.

My life was getting so confusing.

Sunday, November 09, 2003

I Don't Wanna Wear a Sheitel!!

I was in a very bad mood the next morning. I hadn't slept well that night and I was tired and cranky. I kept waking up all night drenched in my sweat and it wasn't pleasant. The doctor had told me that this symptom of cancer would not go away until I started chemo.

It sounds terrible but I was sort of excited for chemo to start. Changing my pajamas three times a night was not a load of fun.

My aunt and uncle took me to get a sheitel from Clyde a wig-maker, Chai Lifeline sent us there, because they were paying for the wig.

Everyone was so excited about getting me this stunning wig, but I was in a bad mood for the rest of the day.

I didn't wanna wear a sheitel! I loved my long hair!

Monday, November 10, 2003

More Sheitlach and Some Sad Things

*M*onday morning I went to school just to get attention.

Actually, I went to speak to my principal about something, but he wasn't there, so I just hung around the teacher's room and let all the teachers kiss me.

Later I had a nice time telling my mother which teachers said which thoughtless things. It was an amazing experience I think every teen should have at least once.

I went home after that and spent most of my morning writing in this journal because my Aunt Blima from London told me to do so, and because Ruchy Perlstein (the neighbor who had sent me to buy those *Perek Shirah* booklets) bought me this adorable Cat in the Hat journal to write in.

She had written the most adorable poem on the first page:

> *Read this tale of up and down,*
> *Will you laugh or cry or frown?*
> *Will you, do you, want this gift?*
> *I bought it for you to give you a lift!*
> *"I'm here to give chizuk; I know just what to say!*
> *I'll call and I'll visit, day after day!"*
> *(Oh NO!!)*
> *Look at me! Look at me now!*
> *I'm getting too many phone calls, I've gotta hang up somehow!*
> *Now Dr. Seuss is put to use,*
> *As you really LET IT LOOSE!*
> *— Happy writing!*

During my writing, my math teacher, Miss Riegler, called to talk to me, and she told me that she was also going through a hard time now. She had a form of diabetes and though it was under control, she knew what it was like to be sick. She said she would love to be there for me if I needed anything. She told me never to hesitate to call her.

She told me a little about what it was like for her to struggle with her illness and then she told me that she was having a hard time finding a *shidduch* because of it. She was fine and knew how to take care of herself, but she said that people were afraid to get involved with someone who had been sick.

I felt so bad for her.

I liked her a lot. She was a young teacher, and she always seemed to be in on the things we students were interested in. She was spunky and on the ball, and there was no getting by her in class. I never would have guessed she had to stick herself for insulin tests every day. She was so ... normal.

It felt good to have someone go through a hard time together with me, but still, I couldn't help wondering, why did so many people have to suffer?

After I hung up with Miss Riegler, Morah Templer called. She wanted to take me out for lunch because she heard I hadn't been eating anything for about three weeks.

The weirdest thing happened when I walked outside. My port got cold.

I was all warm and bundled in my coat, and the port under my skin was still cold. It felt like I had some cold Jell-O stuck somewhere in my chest. I tapped my fingers on it to see if it would move, and it made a loud noise. It was like my own mini drum!

From then on, whenever I got bored, I would tap the port and play some tunes. People said I was immature, but I thought it was cool.

I had to carry a card with me at all times that said that I had a port in me. It was to explain why I beeped when I went through metal detectors.

My mother came home that day with a second cell phone, because it was cheaper to buy a new one than to add minutes to her existing plan. I was happy about that because it meant that I got to use the phone when my mother didn't need it. It made Faigy and my brothers Zevy and Pinny and everyone else so jealous, but it was sad in a way to see my mom with two cell phones, trying to do some work on one, and trying to reach doctors on the other.

Chavy was always short-tempered with me whenever she had to babysit because of my appointments. She had always complained that she did most of the work around the house and that I didn't do half as much as she did. When she was engaged all she could talk about was how I'd have to start helping out more when she wasn't there and that I'd finally see what it was like to be in her shoes. I felt bad that even after she was married, it was because of me that she was still doing most of the work.

Faigy tried to avoid me as much as possible because she was always afraid I was going to tell her or show her something to nauseate her.

Zevy was preparing for his bar mitzvah and he was upset by all the attention I was getting when it was his year to shine. I didn't mean to take it away from him, but it wasn't my fault. I felt so guilty about it and I couldn't even do anything to change it.

My ten-year-old brother Pinny was livid with all the attention I got. He always claimed his sisters ruined his life and I couldn't disagree with him this time.

The other siblings were still a little young to know much, but they all felt it even if they couldn't say exactly what it was that they felt.

It was all my fault.

My grandmother took me to another *sheitelmacher*, Rachelli Cohen, that night, to get another wig. She was such a nice person and was so easy to talk to. She couldn't believe that my grandmother was really a grandmother; she said she looked way too young.

My grandma got really excited about that!

My grandmother wanted to take me back home with her so that I wouldn't have to be around all my siblings all the time and be exposed to so many germs. I told her that I was fine where I was, and the truth is, I don't think my parents would have allowed it anyway.

I was nervous when I went to bed that night because I had an appointment with that New Jersey doctor, Dr. Harris, the next day. I was a little annoyed at having to go and get so many opinions when I was already happy with Dr. Robinson, but like my parents said, when it came to my health, we had to try everything.

The truth is, we were extremely happy with Dr. Robinson, but too many people were telling us about Hackensack University Medical Center, a hospital in New Jersey. Everyone we met had either gone there or knew someone who had been there and said we should at least check it out.

A man from a medical referral agency that we were in contact with tried to convince my parents that even if I could just get in to be under the care of any of the doctors on the team at Hackensack, I would still be in a better environment than in Manhattan. When he got us the appointment with Dr. Harris, the top doctor there, my parents felt that we had to go see what it was about.

Wednesday,
November 12, 2003

Hackensack
and Grad Photos

*W*e had an appointment on Tuesday in the pediatric clinic of Hackensack in New Jersey. The top doctor there, Dr. Harris, didn't usually encourage people to switch doctors, but he did say that if I wanted to make the switch, he would personally accept my case.

We were all pretty worried about my being sick, and we spoke to a woman who was able to do some things and found a couple of *ayin haras* on my name. My cousin Dovid Levy heard about everything going on and wanted to help, so he bought me a *kamiyah* to wear around my neck. We were taking no chances — not with my *ayin haras* or with my doctors.

The clinic in Hackensack was beautiful! It was like a hotel! It took less than an hour to drive there, and there was free parking for patients. The whole area was spacious and cheerful; not at all like the dreary, beeping, and cramped places we had dealt with in the city. This was a modern hospital with an out-of-town flavor.

The staff was also different. If we had to wait, someone would keep us updated on what was going on and how much longer we'd be waiting. It wasn't like in Manhattan, when we kept being told to wait for another five minutes every six hours.

And Dr. Harris was just as nice, if not nicer, than Dr. Robinson! Right away he noticed that my mother called me by my Hebrew name and not by my legal name. He made a note of that and never in all the time that I was under his care did he call me anything but what my family called me.

He also agreed never to call me *Sweetie* or *Honey*, only *Champ*. We compromised on *Sugar* when Dr. Harris offered to call me *Glucose*. My mother told him I liked biology, and it was like our own private joke.

He asked me a load of questions about how I was feeling and if I had any other problems besides my sweats and my weight loss and whatever. I told him I had Obsessive Talking Disorder. He was so quick to smile and tell me he had it too! That sealed the deal for me. I decided I was staying with him.

The hard part of the day was calling Dr. Robinson to tell him that we wanted to switch. He was such a mensch about it though, and said I had to do what was best for me, and he didn't mind — as long as I still invited him to my wedding one day.

I went to school on Wednesday to speak to my principal, and then I ended up staying there for the rest of the day. My principal asked me what I was doing spiritually during my illness to help me learn and grow from the experience, and I said that we were saying *Perek Shirah* and saying a lot of *Tehillim.*

He told me to leave the *Tehillim* to others and to focus on something concrete; a *kabbalah* I could take on for always. He said that he had taken on to become involved in making *shidduchim* because he was not a well man. He said he'd thought of it because in *Tefillas HaShachar,* in "*Ailu Devarim,*" it lists different mitzvos, and *hachnasas kallah*, helping brides, comes between *bikur cholim* and *levayas hameis,* Since *shidduchim* comes between sickness and death, he felt this would save him from harm.

I always knew that my principal was busy with *shidduchim,* but the reason behind it was very moving.

I left his office thinking very deeply about something that I could take upon myself, but to be honest, it was a very hard thing to do. It was something I had think about for a very long time until I came up with something that I felt was half-decent.

I resolved to try and kiss the mezuzah every time I passed through a doorway. I felt that it was Hashem's sign on the door and that as long as I made the effort to reach up to Him, He would hold my hand.

From the minute I walked into class, I was a celebrity. Everyone treated me like some superstar — except for one teacher who gave me some homework to make up for her class. Funny thing was that she had excused Faigy from doing all homework for her periods.

I didn't mind the people crowding around me during recess — it was fun seeing other girls become jealous over all the attention showered on me! I did end up getting annoyed at some of the stupid questions the girls asked, though. One kid wanted to know if I was really going to come to school bald.

Of course I didn't blame them for being so curious; they

didn't know what to say, but a little bit of brains would have been greatly appreciated.

My mother arranged for me to take graduation pictures that night. I had the idea because I started thinking that I would probably still be bald by yearbook pictures the next year, and I didn't want to take my pictures in a sheitel, so I asked the school if I could take them now.

I have to say that my school was pretty amazing the whole time I was sick. Of course, nothing is perfect, and there were plenty of times I was annoyed with teachers and classmates, but in general my school handled the whole thing very well. They were exceptionally accommodating and understanding of the situation. The teachers looked out for Faigy, too, and helped both of us so much with whatever we needed.

The teacher in charge of graduation and yearbook gave me a graduation gown to wear for pictures and set up an appointment with the school's photographer.

I got the cutest haircut and I looked even better once my mother finished putting on my makeup. I put on the graduation gown for the pictures, and I felt so adult every time I looked in the mirror.

The man who usually took the graduation pictures for my school told us to come over to his house where he set up a special shoot for us in his basement. He said he had never done that before but was glad to help us out.

He spent a lot of time getting me to sit right and smile right and making sure I got the best pictures possible to choose from. He even wanted my mother to get into the pictures with me. After he finished the grad photos, he took more just for fun.

They all came out beautiful, but when I looked back at them it was amazing to see what chemo had done to me. A few weeks later I looked completely different. Even after I got well, I never regained that same look. People say my face changed entirely over the course of that year.

That night I almost forgot that I was sick. I had so much fun taking pictures and smiling until my face felt about to break in half. The *chesed* that man showed us in his basement photo shoot that night was a tremendous inspiration, and we couldn't thank him enough for what he did.

Thursday, November 13, 2003

More Scans and a Big Schlep

*T*hursday was a huge schlep. My father came along to Hackensack to meet my new doctor and check out the place. When we got there, I found out that I had an echocardiogram and a pulmonary-function test scheduled that day in addition to meeting the doctor.

We did the echo first. A really nice technician was there, and she explained to me that this test was to make sure that my heart continued functioning properly even while on chemo. Some of the chemo I was going to get might have an impact on my heart, so they had to monitor me very carefully.

She smeared an icky gel on me and put a probe on to monitor my heartbeat and blood flow. I almost hurt my neck as I twisted it to see the screen.

It was quite cool, actually. I heard funny noises as my heart pumped blood and I saw red and blue blood going in and out of its chambers.

It wasn't a bad test except that it was cold and uncomfortable lying there in an ICU gown.

We then went to meet Dr. Harris. He had finished going through all my reports and viewing all my CT scan slides that I had taken in NYU. Now he was ready to outline my chemo protocol.

I agreed to go onto a clinical research thingy which meant that if all went well, I would get a lower total amount of chemo than was usually given to Hodgkin's patients.

Hodgkin's patients were usually given six to eight rounds of chemo. They were first given three, then tested to see if they were clean, and then given another three or more rinse rounds of chemo.

Patients used to be bombarded with loads of chemo just to get everything out of the system. But the more the disease was studied, the more they began wondering if they couldn't pinpoint a more precise amount of meds per patient. So that's where all these experimental studies came into play. They started slowly lowering the dosage, watching carefully for the results. I was more than happy to volunteer for science and walk away from my chemo all that much sooner.

This new study wanted to start testing patients to see if they were clean after only two rounds of chemo, rather than three. If they were clean, they'd get only two rinse rounds. If they still weren't clean, they'd go right back onto the regular treatment of six or so rounds and then some radiation.

This new treatment had another great thing to it besides

less chemo. If all went well, I might be one of the random patients in the study chosen not to have radiation. That seemed like a big plus for me.

My parents and the doctor left the decision all up to me, and I told them that I would be part of the study.

After all that was decided, I had to run to a pulmonary-function test, which was an intensive breathing test that left me very sore after forty-five minutes of making myself crazy dizzy, huffing and puffing into a tube.

Dr. Harris then met with us again and went through all the medications that I was going to be taking during chemo. He legally had to explain all the side effects to me. It took forever and we were all so tired, but I was glad to get it done. It gave me an idea of what I was about to face.

He told me that each cycle, or round, of chemo was going to consist of three weeks. In the first week I would take three consecutive days of chemotherapy, and then I would have a few days off. In the second week I would only have one day of chemo, and then I would have the rest of the week and the next week off, too.

It sounded okay, but I soon learned that there was no such thing as a day off. Nausea, emergencies, and tons of scans took care of any extra days we originally thought we had.

Before we left Hackensack, we noticed that the gas in New Jersey was much cheaper than gas in New York. It was $1.49 a gallon, while at home it was almost $2.00. My mother took advantage and filled up her tank even though it was still about half-full. That was the best part of our day.

We got home at 7:30.

I had a sheitel appointment that night, but I had to cancel it. Chavy had a family *simchah* from Eli's side and she needed the time to be a new wife. She couldn't be busy taking care of my siblings every night. Faigy was none too happy about babysitting in her place. She was crazy about keeping up her marks in school, and taking care of everyone was making it really hard on her.

She was also upset because her Bop-It pen broke and she wanted a new one. My mother offered to write to the company for her and she was slightly happier.

I wanted to help out too, but I was so tired that by 8 p.m. I was dead asleep in my clothing.

Motza'ei Shabbos, November 15, 2003

First Life Lesson About Pajamas

I managed to convince my mother to send my two-year-old brother Yitzy away for Shabbos so that she could have a rest. So my aunt and uncle came for him a couple of hours before the *z'man*. The other kids went away too, and even our regular Shabbos guests didn't come that week.

It was only my parents, my three-year-old sister Nechama, my four-year-old brother Shmully, and myself.

Faigy was home too, but she was having a Sophomore Shabbos kind of thing where a bunch of girls slept over in our basement and pretty much hibernated there all Shabbos, only emerging to run off to school for their scheduled program.

We didn't see or hear them … much.

Friday night I was pretty upset at them because I wanted to go to sleep and I woke up drenched in sweat, and when I finally changed and got back into bed again, I heard my sister and her friends make their noisy entrance. My room was right over the front hallway and I heard everything,

I was just dozing off again when I heard some more knocking at the door.

By this time Faigy and her friends were making such a racket in the basement that they probably couldn't hear the knocking. So I had to get out of bed and open the door myself.

I wasn't wearing my contacts, but when I looked out the peephole I saw two girls standing there. I was annoyed. Why couldn't my sister's friends just walk home together and come in all at once?

I opened the door, in my pajamas and robe, and surprise, surprise — the two girls standing there were not Faigy's friends. They were Miss Riegler and her friend.

I learned a life lesson about pajamas then: They are not meant to open the door in. It can be quite embarrassing sometimes.

Once I got over my shock, I invited them in and we had a great time, my tiredness all but forgotten. As we were laughing about something, my sister's friends came upstairs and on a dare, one of the girls began kissing my feet as the others laughed.

When she was done, she turned to Miss Riegler and said that part of her dare was to kiss her shoes too. It was dark, and she had no idea who she was talking to.

When Miss Riegler told her that in eleventh-grade Math class she would remind the girl of whose toes she had just tried to kiss, the kid almost started crying.

It was worth being woken up so many times that night just to see the look on the girls' faces when they realized they were standing in front of their future Math teacher in pajamas.

Seems like they learned a lesson about pajamas that night too!

Sunday,
November 16, 2003

I'm So Pretty!

D evoiry Parnes was my friend since I had switched schools in 4th grade. She was the first one to share her markers with me, and I shared my snack. Since then, we did almost everything together. We studied with each other, passed notes in class, and wore the same high ponytails with big scrunchies until they were way out of style.

We were there for each other through so many different hardships. I was there when Devoiry's parents got divorced and now she planned to be there for me when I needed her.

She was the one who begged the attendance lady to let some girls come and take me out to Macy's to get all painted up at the Lancôme counter. She told the teacher that I was so pale and that I was really miserable to look at without some color, and that was why I needed four girls to take me to the mall.

The girls were all thrilled with the unexpected day off from school and we were all really excited to be allowed to practice our favorite hobby — shopping!

We ran into a bit of a problem with buying mascara because if my eyelashes were going to fall out there would be no point in spending all that money on it.

The woman behind the counter was so nice to me. My friends told her that I was sick and she started crying and she told me that her aunt had had cancer the year before and she felt so bad, so she gave me a big bag full of free samples and a big hug, and she told me to get better.

I got a little depressed later when my friends were busy shopping in the hair accessories aisle. They didn't mean to make me feel bad; they just weren't thinking.

I was sitting off to a side watching them fool around with hair clips, when Miss Riegler turned up. She seemed to have a GPS tracking device on me.

She was shopping with her friend, too. She said that she needed to shop for shoes to get her mind off *shidduchim*. While she was looking at a pair of shoes that was way too pointy for my taste, her friend told me that Miss Riegler had come very close to becoming engaged but the boy's side broke it off at the last minute.

I felt so bad for her. She was young and spunky and so much fun, and no one that nice should have had to go through something that tough. I couldn't figure out what the boy's problem was. Miss Riegler was so special.

I almost asked her to give me a ride home because I was bored shopping for headbands I couldn't even wear, but I stayed with my friends in the end and had a good time.

I bought a nice sweater for myself and a matching one for Faigy, (which meant that Chavy was upset that I didn't get her one, too, and then my eight-year-old sister Ruchie decided she wanted one as well ...) and it was a nice outing in the end.

A couple of people called me that night to give me "*chizuk*." What they all said was nice, but it sounded a little empty. It's always so easy to say something inspiring when it's not you going through the hard time.

I heard some very interesting things that night. There were people who had either very little tact or very little brains, even if they might have had very big hearts.

"Hashem chose you to be sick because it gives a wake-up call to everyone who knows you and no one else knows everyone that you know."

And, "Hashem loves you soooooooooooo much and that's why He's doing this to you!"

And, "Hashem is sending you a message and you need to think about what it is He wants to tell you ...."

You know what I did? I disconnected my phone.

Though I got annoyed with people easily, a lot of *chesed* was being done all around me. I went over to Meira's house for some breathing room, just to air out, and her family surprised me by having printed up some really neat cards with a nice *tefillah* on them for me to give out, in the hope that with people saying this *tefillah* I would have a complete *refuah*.

Later, my father showed me a rubber stamp he created with my name on it so that whenever he lent out money from his *gemach*, he could stamp the check with my name, so that in the *zechus* of the loan, I should get well.

I was kind of lonely that night because even with all the phone calls and stuff I didn't think anyone could understand how I felt.

Miss Riegler called later to ask me how my day at the mall turned out and it felt nice talking to someone who was having tough times of her own. She was able to sympathize with all the dumb things people were saying to me. She gave me some of her own *chizuk*, but it was easier to take. One of her best friends had gotten engaged that day and she was taking it a little hard. She was in pain like I was, and if she could live by the words she told me that night, then so could I.

It was a lot easier to take it from someone who knew rather than from someone who was just making me her *chesed* (however much appreciated) for the day.

Monday, November 17, 2003

Day Before Chemo

Monday morning started off awful. The babysitter didn't show up and we had to take Yitzy to the clinic with us. We left the other kids with a neighbor to put on the school bus.

We were running so late, but once we got to the clinic everything calmed down. My brother went straight to the playroom while I got weighed in and had my blood pressure taken.

I had to take some blood tests but my nurse was so nice that I didn't mind her at all. Her name was Jess and she was wearing two different earrings! One of the earrings was just a sterilized safety pin stuck through her ear. She seemed like a character.

She kept me laughing as she drew my blood and mentioned that her son was a senior marketing agent for Gap stores. I had been searching all over for a specific sweatshirt that had been discontinued for a while and asked her if her son could possibly find one for me. She made no promises, but it was cool to know someone who had a connection to my favorite clothing chain.

Jess left the IV line in my hand for the CT scan I needed to do later and I went to take an electrocardiogram. It was different than an echocardiogram in that instead of the gooky mess they used on me last time, they stuck stickers all over me and attached wires to them in order to monitor my heart rate.

I didn't even have to wear a gown, and I was out of there in less than twenty minutes.

Then my mother and I ran halfway around the building to find the CT-scan area. It was beautiful. The waiting room was all wood and glass and armchairs. It felt like a hotel lounge.

The people working there were amazing too. They came out to tell us that they were an hour behind schedule so that we'd be updated and not annoyed and impatient. It was so different from in Manhattan where everything was "only another five minutes" for the next six hours.

I needed to take this scan because the other one was outdated by this time. Dr. Harris wanted to make sure that he knew exactly where all my lumps were and if they had spread before starting chemo the next day.

The chest x-ray that I had to go for next was by far the easiest thing I ever did. I just had to stand in front of a machine for all of two seconds so that they could x-ray my chest. The technician told me that it was really safe, but she was going to stand in a far corner behind a big screen.

I put her on the spot by asking her if it was so safe, why she was hiding all the way over there? She was a little embarrassed and I enjoyed every minute of it. I really can be a pain, can't I?

Back at the clinic I was given a special numbing cream called Emla. Jess told me to rub it over my port site the next morning so that I'd be numb when they stuck me there to start my chemotherapy.

I had a great day, and when I got home I got my wig cut and done and Chavy even came over to try it on! She was jealous of how gorgeous it looked. She helped me put it on and take it off a hundred times and showed me how to take care of my sheitel and how to make it sit right on my head. I was lucky to have a sister who knew it all.

Chemo

My mother woke me up early Tuesday morning with a gallon of water. She said I had to drink all of it before we left to Hackensack. The nurses told her that the more I drank before chemo, the less nauseous I would be.

I was already feeling nausea from nervousness and drinking nonstop made me feel even sicker. I tried to stop drinking, but my mother kept refilling my bottle and made me down it all.

I even made up a little song about it as we were stuck in traffic and I had to take still another sip of the stuff.

"I'm a little camel, short and stout,
Pour some more water into my mouth.

Before you take chemo, you just can't stop,
So give me water till I pop!"

Obviously, the tune was "I'm a little teapot ...."

In the rush that morning, I had forgotten all about the Emla cream. I didn't numb my port site before driving down to the clinic, so it hurt a little when the nurse stuck the needle into me.

I was asked if I wanted to be accessed with a big needle or a small one. What a stupid question. With someone of my heightened intelligence and maturity and sensitivity, I chose the small one.

I was in the middle of contemplating why anyone would even bother creating a big needle if a small one was good enough, when my IV line started beeping loudly. The nurses came running and fixed it, but almost right away it began beeping again.

I soon found out the reason for the bigger needle. It was made to fit my type of port better. The small one didn't flow as well into the catheter I had.

I had to be de-accessed and then stuck again, this time, with the BIG needle.

Jess, the nurse with the safety-pin earring, took me into another room to redo the IV line. I climbed onto the table and was listening to her talk while sterilizing her needle and I have no idea how or why it happened, but I suddenly burst into tears. I rolled over and buried my face into my hoodie and cried like a two-year-old.

I think Jess wasn't expecting all that from me, but she was wonderful. She held my hand and let me cry until I was ready to go back and meet my mother in the infusion room.

The infusion room was a large room with lots of overstuffed blue armchairs that gave the ilussion of some privacy. All the outpatient kids did chemo together in the infusion room, but we didn't have to stay there. If we felt well enough, we were allowed to wheel our IV poles down the hall into the playroom or the teen room.

I loved the teen room. It had its own jukebox, arcade games, football table, and huge bookshelf with lots of stuff to read. There were also some bright couches and chairs to relax on. My favorite part of the room was that everything in it was free. It didn't cost anything to play the arcades or the jukebox. It was really cool.

At first I thought that I'd never sit in the infusion room, but very quickly I learned that there is a reason chemo Isn't a picnic. I ended up feeling so awful most of the time that just opening my eyes made me nauseous. Going to the teen room was usually not even one of my options.

The first day of my cycle was really long. It was about eight straight hours of chemo. My mother and I watched some movies together and then a friend of hers who lived nearby came over and brought us lunch.

She called ahead and asked me what I wanted to eat and I asked for my all-time favorite — sesame chicken.

Years later, the smell, taste, sight, and even thought of sesame chicken makes me ill. I had forgotten all about my friend Etty's warning, and ate something I liked while on chemo. I never, ever, want to eat sesame chicken again!

Back to chemo. All the time I was on medication I had to go to the bathroom about every fifteen minutes or so. I was on hydration to minimize the effects of the chemo and to prevent dehydration. I hated going because I was too sick to get up so often and schlep my IV pole after me into such a small cubicle.

The first couple of times I went to the bathroom I ended up getting tangled in all the IV lines and somehow tied myself to the sink. I considered calling a nurse to untangle me, but every time I was about to do that, I just needed the bathroom again, so it worked out kind of well.

I finally got myself free by turning the knob on the sink and the door at the same time. I wheeled my pole back to my seat, and had enough time to think about sitting down before I needed to go back again.

I was doing okay until they gave me Cytoxin. I literally felt it making me sick as it went through my IV line. My mother said that every time I got Cytoxin, my eyes glazed over and she was able to see me become nauseous. If there was a picture to capture the essence of nausea, I was it.

We filled up on gas at the Sunoco station right near the highway, and realized that it was getting more expensive; it was already up to $1.52 a gallon. But it was still cheaper than at home, so we told the attendant to "fill'er up" and then made the long drive back.

I remember feeling awful all the way home, but not much else. When I got home, I gave back all the sesame chicken I had eaten for lunch, and then some.

When I was sick, pomegranate juice wasn't being sold in every Shop Rite around the country, so my aunt made me some from scratch. She claimed it had tons of nutrients that my body needed during chemo. My parents forced me to drink it, but I was too sick to appreciate it.

The nice part of the juice was the utter coolness of throwing up purple. That was the best part of my day. The worst part was knowing I had to do it all again the next day.

Friday, November 21, 3003

Rest of the Week on Chemo

Miri came along to chemo the next day. Ayala met us in Hackensack where her brother was coming in for some tests that day. It was great in that when I wasn't feeling so well, Ayala was able to keep Miri company and explain to her everything that was going on.

Ayala had been shocked when Miri and I called her to tell her that I was the one going to a hematologist. She was so upset that someone else close to her was going through cancer; but she was still very cool about it all, and helped out a lot by explaining all those foreign terms to me.

During the infusion, Dr. Harris came to see me and said that he'd heard from Jess that I had cried the day before. I told him that I was very embarrassed and that I didn't mean to cry and that I didn't even know why I did it and how it happened.

Dr. Harris thought I was a little crazy because all he had come to tell me was that he was relieved that I was finally admitting that it was okay to be scared and upset. He said that he was worried when I was so happy all the time. It wasn't expected of me and it definitely wasn't normal, so I didn't have to pretend to be all strong all the time.

He assured me that it was okay to cry when I needed to, and he was so nice about it all; that conversation made me want to cry all over again.

He was such a great guy. A real mentch.

I slept for most of the day, and felt so much better on the way home than I did the day before. I didn't speak much in the car, but Miri didn't need me to. She was very awed by the whole day and was happy and relieved to have seen all that. It made everything more realistic, but also less scary to her. She was now able to picture exactly what I did all day in the hospital, and she knew that they were taking care of me, and even though I was sick and tired and cranky, I was still the same friend I always was to her.

I went right to bed when I got home, and then woke up at 5:30. I thought it was 5:30 a.m., but then I heard all the noise downstairs and realized I had only slept for about three hours.

I went down to the kitchen where Zevy and Pinny were doing some comical imitations of their teachers and of us, but laughing made my head hurt, so I went right back up to bed and slept until I had to get up for chemo on Tuesday.

Tuesday's chemo took only three hours. I got a teddy bear and a jester doll that came with a book called *The Jester Has*

Lost his Jingle, by David Saltzman. Sue Daniels, the child-life specialist there, read it to me. It was a kid's book, but had a much deeper meaning. It was about a jester who made the discovery that laughter and cheer really come from within and that we would never find true happiness until we learned to stop relying on others for happiness instead of on ourselves.

I came home and slept all day and only got up later because we were ordering clothing from Land's End and I wanted some stuff too. Faigy was getting some really cute sweaters and when I wanted to order some, we realized that I had lost a lot of weight over the week. I was getting to be a smaller size than Faigy. I liked being thin, but ordering a junior's size twelve was a little weird.

As we were on the phone ordering, I leafed through their catalog and found a delicious fleece blanket that wasn't too expensive. Before chemo started, my parents bought me a throw blanket to take around with me in the hospital, but it was very heavy and bulky, so I didn't like taking it along. Faigy and my little sister Ruchie were fighting over who got to keep it now that I didn't want it.

I showed the other blanket to my mother, who asked the salesperson on the phone if the blanket I was looking at was lightweight. She explained she wanted it for a cancer patient who wanted to take it with her to chemo and to the hospital but didn't want to schlep anything heavy.

The sales rep was so nice and said that it was light enough to take anywhere, and that if it was for a cancer patient she wanted to give us a discount. She spoke to her supervisor and they gave it to me for less. I was so impressed with the kind of people who worked there. Land's End always says how great they are at customer service, but here they really outdid themselves.

This blanket I was going to get now was blue on one side

and red on the other. Of course, I always slept with the red side facing up. I had more than enough of blue with all the blue shirts I was wearing to the hospital.

Who ever heard of a sixteen year old with a security blanket? Miri said it was part of my Maturiosity.

Friday morning, my mother's brother Shimi came along to the hospital to donate blood for me. He and I were both A+ blood type, so we wanted his blood to be on reserve in my name in case I ever needed a blood transfusion. My mother had A-, but for some reason they didn't want her to give for me. I always thought that a negative could give to a positive, but not the opposite way around. Whatever. I wasn't the one who made the rules. I think the doctors just thought that if there was enough A+ blood to go around, why even take A-?

Since she wasn't able to give me blood, my mother looked for something else to do, so she learned how to give me an injection!

Because my white blood count was very low, I was prescribed a GCSF shot to make my bones produce more. The nurses made my mother practice on a plum before she gave it to me, and she did a great job.

I was used to getting stuck about ten times a day, so the needle in itself didn't bother me much, but the fluid inside it burned terribly. After a few tries, we figured out that if my mother pinched my arm tightly when she inserted the needle, it hurt a lot less.

My mother was told to alternate the shots between my left and right arms and then legs because the Neupogen, the fluid inside the shots, could burn me if I got it too often in the same place.

On coming home, we came into a dining room full of helium balloons. A family I babysat for sent three. The Landers from across the street sent one with a box of candy, and my cousins sent one with a really ugly picture of me scanned onto it.

Morah Templer sent over some cake that sent all the adults within a two-mile radius into seventh heaven, but I was not interested.

It was so weird. I looked at food, willed myself to eat it, but I had no appetite. I wasn't nauseated by food; I just had no feel for it. Most dieting girls would love to feel the way I felt, but I found it sort of annoying. I would walk into the kitchen, go into the pantry, open the fridge, and look at the food, over and over again. I knew I had to eat something, but I wasn't in the mood for anything. It drove me nuts.

Chemo Makes My Life a Mess

After Shabbos we had a bit of a problem with the GCSF shot. Each dosage was given in its own small glass bottle and each bottle was only about half-full. In order to fill the needle, we needed to turn the bottle upside-down, stick the needle through the wire top of the bottle, and draw up the medicine. My mother couldn't figure out how to get the liquid up into the needle without getting any air into the syringe.

We had to call our pharmacist friend to come over and help us out. He showed us how to draw the syringe up properly, and he even brought me some thinner needles as a gift. He told my brothers never to touch my Neupogen bottles because each and every capsule was worth three hundred dollars.

I could see dollar signs flashing in Pinny's eyes as Dovid, the nine-year-old genius, told him that we had about $3,000 of Neupogen sitting in our fridge.

Later, Chavy took me and Faigy and Ruchie to the mall. It was way past Ruchie's bedtime, but she insisted on coming and my mother made us take her along. Faigy bought a bunch of clothing and Ruchie bought everything she saw that was pink, and I saw double all night.

I had noticed that I'd been having blurry vision for a few days already, and on Sunday it didn't get any better. Not only couldn't I see, but I also had the most awful mouth sores on my tongue, inside my cheeks, and down my throat. In addition, I was also on a steroid called Prednisone that was making my cheeks look blotchy and horrible.

I felt the way I looked.

We had a camp reunion that night that I felt I had to go to. It was a good thing that I did go, because the camp had no program planned. Instead, everyone sat around me for three hours and asked stupid questions about being sick till my mother rescued me and came to pick me up.

I got a lot of compliments that night. My face had thinned out a lot and it made my eyes look huge. I looked like one of those Precious Moments characters, except I was dark-haired and hazel-eyed instead of blonde and blue. And unlike the Precious Moments dolls, I didn't have those round cherubic cheeks. Chemo was taking care of that.

Being a sudden celebrity got on my nerves just a little bit. Many of the girls who were obsessed with me all night were the ones who were too cool to be seen with me in camp. I guess I became cool enough for everyone as soon as I was diagnosed with a scary illness.

I thought it so sad that despite my talents and personality, having cancer was what made me so popular now.

I begged my parents to let me go to school on Monday, but my father didn't think it was a good idea. I had spent all weekend complaining that my bones were sore and hurting and that I was seeing double, and he was worried about sending me off to class.

Silly me, I begged hard enough to change my father's mind and the next morning found me wearing my uniform and walking to school.

I sat through the first period *parashah* lesson but didn't take any notes. I spent the time catching up on my cancer diary. The class was reviewing for a test and I was living it up by not caring a bit about school work. I was keeping up with Regents subjects like Math and Science and English and History, but other than those, I didn't care a lick about my grades.

I was enjoying being at the center of attention when my mother called the school and left a message for me to meet her a few blocks away, because she was coming to pick me up and rush me to Hackensack. She had called Dr. Harris about my blurry vision, and he wanted me to come in pronto because he was worried that it might be a bad reaction to some of the chemo.

Dr. Harris wanted me to see a Dr. Thomas, the neurologist in Hackensack, but he wasn't in the clinic that day. After some debating, I was sent to another doctor twenty minutes away. My mother and I had a short wait of about two hours, and then I did a bunch of tests that made me insanely dizzy.

At the end, I learned that everyone has a blind spot in their vision, and that the doctors got lens solution free from different companies who want to promote their products, and that the blurriness was a reaction from the GCSF shot. It was nothing to worry about except a wasted day.

Wednesday, November 26, 2003

So This Is Why They Hate Chemo

*M*y mother had to go back to work on Tuesday, so her friend, Mrs. Kohn, offered to go along to Hackensack with me. Mrs. Kohn didn't drive, so we arranged to get a ride with a Chai Lifeline volunteer.

My infusion took only half-an-hour. I got some hydration and then a chemo called Vincristine. After the infusion, my port was flushed with Heparin and it left an icky taste in my mouth.

After I was de-accessed, I met with Dr. Thomas, the neurologist Dr. Harris had wanted me to meet the day before.

He checked my eyes and told me I was just fine and that my shoes were very cool.

The day was turning out great except that I didn't like the sandwich my mother had packed for my lunch.

I was home by lunchtime and in bed with a migraine twenty minutes later. I tried to sleep but I couldn't. After tossing and turning in bed for four hours, I went downstairs to where my family was eating supper and I made it just in time to open the door for the UPS man who was delivering my Land's End stuff.

I was so excited with my new blanket that I spread it out on the kitchen floor and went right to sleep.

My parents were worried because my headache wasn't going away. They wanted to take me into Hackensack to check it out, but then all that codeine I took began to work and I felt much better. Everyone relaxed, and I slept in my own bed that night.

I woke up Wednesday morning and decided to start my day. I just about made it to the bathroom before I fainted.

That was the end of my day.

I called my mother at work to tell her that I was on the floor and didn't know how I got there and that I couldn't get up without getting dizzy again. I was so thankful to my brother Yitzy because he had dropped the cordless phone on the bathroom floor when he was done playing with it that morning. It was right near me when I fell, and I was able to call my parents right away.

I was told to get back into bed, but every time I tried, I blacked out again. In the end I stayed where I was until my mother literally picked me up and rushed me to the hospital.

Right away I was strapped onto a stretcher and had a line put into my hand for hydration and antibiotics. The doctors didn't want to use my port because they were afraid that I might have an infection there.

I was freezing cold, and whenever I had a conscious moment, I asked for another blanket. But no matter what they piled on me, I still shook. I was hot with a fever, but I couldn't get warm. I lay like that for three hours because just as they had wheeled me into the emergency room, our insurance company called to inform us that they were stopping my insurance coverage.

They had just realized that they didn't want to cover patients treated outside New York. They could have noticed this for an entire month, but they decided to drop us at the exact time we needed them the most.

As I was being taken care of by the medical staff, my parents tried to get me onto another insurance plan. I didn't know what was worse; how sick I felt, or how guilty I felt for being the cause of such a mess.

Once my insurance was taken care of, I met a doctor I decided that I wasn't going to like. She told me that I was most probably going to have to stay in the hospital until Friday afternoon. I was so upset, I said something nasty, and she told me to grow up and not be such a baby.

Then she decided to be nice and she told me that because I was sick, Make a Wish Foundation was going to give me anything I wanted. She asked me what I wanted most in the whole world.

I told her very seriously that I wanted an Uzi submachine gun.

She asked me whatever for.

I smiled sweetly and told her that an Uzi would be very helpful in getting rid of people and doctors who were annoying me.

She said that Make a Wish would never give kids with a temper like mine a gun. I told her that it was totally fine; if it were up to me, I would never give people with her bad bedside manner a license to practice medicine.

The doctor got angry and left the room.

I didn't mind in the least.

I was wheeled from the clinic to the 6th floor of the Rocklin Building where all the inpatient kids stayed overnight.

My father stayed with me as I tried to go to sleep. I soon found that sleep was the last thing a hospital is good for. Nurses woke me up every four hours to take my vital signs and give me medicines. To me it seemed like I was being awakened up every four hours just to take a sleeping pill.

I didn't like the hospital very much.

Motza'ei Shabbos, November 29, 2003

Shabbos in the Hospital

My father left the hospital Thursday morning as soon as my grandfather came to take his place. My grandfather read his paper while I slept. When I woke up, my mother's brother, Yitzchok Meir, and his wife, Suri, had just arrived to take over my grandfather's shift.

Even with people around me all day, I was still miserable in the hospital, attached to an IV the whole time. By the time Friday rolled around I was downright depressed. I was down and lethargic, but I tried to smile and pretend I was fine so that the doctor would let me go home that afternoon.

My act may have fooled the doctor, but my blood counts didn't. She told me there was no way I was leaving the ward in time for Shabbos. My white blood counts were very low and I had a fever running. It seemed likely that I would have to stay in the hospital until Monday.

If I hadn't been feeling so horrid, I might have punched her.

I hadn't taken a shower since Tuesday night and I felt dirty and itchy. I begged to go home just so I could take a shower and promised to come back after. My nurse laughed and directed me down the hallway where there was a shower stall I could use. She asked me if I wanted help and I told her she could help by guarding the unlocked door while I showered.

I was unhooked from the IV, but not de-accessed. I had to take a shower with one hand covering my port site with a washcloth. I used my other hand to hold on to a bar at the side of the stall to keep me from losing my balance. I was so weak, I could barely stand up without fainting. I realized after a minute or two that I didn't have any hands left to wash with.

The nurse knocked on the door to ask if I was sure I didn't need help, and with all the dignity I had left to me, I refused her services.

As I was standing under the showerhead trying to figure out my next move, I noticed long strands of hair on the floor of the shower. I was nauseated by taking a shower in a dirty stall until I realized that the hair flowing down the drain was mine.

I let go of my port to wash my hair, and a whole bunch of it just came away without any resistance. I quickly took the elastic band I had around my wrist and put my hair into a ponytail. I was very shaken.

After the shower I returned to my room not really feeling any cleaner because I was full of hair and hadn't been able to soap myself very well without the use of my hands.

I met my mother in the room and asked for a comb so that I could make my hair look at least half decent. As I began to untangle my knots, more and more hair fell into the sink. I finally gave up and again pulled it into a loose ponytail.

My parents were not about to leave me alone over Shabbos, so Chavy and Eli slept over at my parents' house and made Shabbos for the rest of the kids while my parents found a way to be with me. I felt really guilty, but I was so lonely and depressed.

Right before Shabbos, while I was moping in bed, an adorable woman popped by to say hello. She said she was on the way to where she was staying for Shabbos, and she had heard of me through some *chesed* organization and she couldn't wait to meet me. She had told her husband to wait in the car and not breathe until she came back.

Her name was Miriam Katz and she ran an organization called "Caring for Kids." She ran around to schools to talk about how to treat kids with illnesses and how to talk to them, etc. She also brought me a stunning pendant on a chain that she liked to give to all her "patients," and then she ran down to check on her husband before he ran out of air, promising that she'd be back to get to know me another day.

After Miriam left, I got a huge package from the Hackensack gift shop: a teddy bear attached to about ten helium balloons. A few friends had chipped in, hoping to cheer me up, and they sure did.

My parents were rushing to set everything up for their stay in the hospital, and the preparations took until my mother had to light Shabbos *licht.* My mother cried when she lit the candles and said that in all the years she was married, she had never welcomed Shabbos not dressed in her Shabbos clothing.

Of course, people are usually dressed for Shabbos by the time they light candles, but do they ever really think about it?

I cried too, but I wasn't sure if I was crying because my mother was sad or because I was just moody.

The nurses were telling me that unless I put some food in my belly, they were not going to send me home for a year. They scared me into eating some of the Shabbos meal, but I really had no appetite. I lay on the bed and watched my parents eat and sing *zemiros* on the floor.

As they were eating the soup, the nurses brought me a present. It was a pint of my Uncle Shimi's blood.

I was scared to get a blood transfusion, but the nurses promised me that I would like it. They were right! The blood felt warm as it dripped into me and it felt awesome. As the infusion continued, I felt energized and gained an appetite for everything I hadn't eaten in the last two weeks. My white lips became visibly pink again and I asked for food.

After this first transfusion, I began to ask for blood when I knew I needed it. It made such a difference in the way I felt.

At 4:00 in the morning my vital signs were taken and I still had a fever. That meant I couldn't go home for at least another two days. They wanted me to be fever-free for at least a full twenty-four hours before sending me home.

I was so depressed then that I began crying. My mother sat down on my bed while I sobbed and she tried to run a hand through my hair. Because I hadn't been able to brush it properly, it was a bit tangled and as my mother's fingers caught in my hair, a huge hank of it came away in her hands.

She looked as sad as I felt. We all knew that chemotherapy made people's hair fall out, but no one told us how creepy it would be. It was the oddest thing to walk outside and see and feel my hair blow away in the wind. I still get the shivers thinking about it.

Shabbos day was pretty boring. I was feeling well enough to take a walk down the ward. At the end of the hallway I found a playroom where there was a little boy playing Nintendo. He told me his name was Carl and that he spent every weekend in the hospital visiting his sister, who was a leukemia patient. He was playing video games as his sister was getting a blood transfusion.

He told me exactly what it felt like to be a sibling of a sick kid, and he made me feel sorry for him and guilty about what I was causing my siblings to feel.

When it came time to eat the meal, my mother ran down to the Clergy office where she had kept our cholent overnight. Our neighbors, the Landers, had prepared a slow cooker full of cholent so that we could have a real Shabbos meal even in the hospital. We couldn't keep it in my room, so the nurses offered to take it over to the Chaplain's office for us.

My mother came back empty-handed. It seems that the secretary there had turned off our cooker because she decided it looked like it was ready, and she didn't want it to get overcooked.

Try explaining to a non-Jewish woman what potato kugel tastes like after it's cooked overnight.

My mother found it hard that her Shabbos wasn't going as planned no matter how hard she tried to make it work, but I assured her that I had no appetite anyway, and that I was just glad they were there with me.

I had a constant stomachache that I named David, and a headache called Louis. My IV pole was Steve, because our family knew someone by that name who was a real drip.

One nurse, Eva, used to walk in and ask how David and Louis were doing before she even checked my vital signs.

My parents left my grandfather in charge after Shabbos. I took his newspaper away after he fell asleep, and I read all the comics. Then I asked for morphine and I was out like a light.

Going Home From the Hospital

One of my counselors from the previous summer in camp asked me if I wanted her to keep me company in the hospital. Chanie got a ride in with my mother Sunday morning and she kept trying to put me to bed all day.

We schmoozed for a little, but because of my mouth sores, it hurt to talk. Chanie was just getting herself a book to read when a woman knocked on our door and asked to come in.

She was a frum woman who said that she lived about a fifteen-minute drive from the hospital and liked to come and visit Jewish patients in the children's ward. She brought her son along to do some magic tricks for me, and she and her boy stayed for about an hour. Chanie hinted to them that I was really tired and they finally left.

I really wished she would have asked the nurses before coming up to my room. I wasn't up to visitors. When she left I cried because I was so tired and miserable. I was embarrassed by how awful I looked and that total strangers came to see me when I looked and felt so bad. She and her son were trying to do *chesed*, but I didn't feel any better.

Chesed was so great, but some people didn't get it. Just because I wasn't doing anything in the hospital, it didn't mean that anyone could just walk in at any time and decide I needed to be kept busy all afternoon.

Chanie was just telling the nurse's station not to forward any calls or visitors to me for a while so that I could rest, when my Aunt Raizy and Uncle Moshe came to visit.

The nice part about having some more unexpected visitors was that they were people I was comfortable enough to cry in front of. I used my new audience to vent about my day and what it felt like in the hospital, and then they left, taking Chanie with them.

I was finally on my own.

When I woke up from napping, I asked my nurse if I could have some codeine for Louis, went to sleep for another hour, spoke to Miss Riegler on the phone, and ate some food that two of my father's friends drove an hour to bring all the way to me.

I had no fever that night and after the blood transfusion I felt so much better, so my night was peaceful. Morning came, and my white counts were up from 0.8 to 1 so I was allowed to go home.

I weighed 97 lbs, but it wasn't enough to worry about medically because I hadn't yet lost ten percent of my original body weight. But it was enough to worry about as a teenager! I was slipping out of all my clothes. Everything was too large. I found it so amazing what a big difference ten pounds made to my skirts.

My fingertips were driving me crazy because they felt as if they were covered in plastic. Dr. Harris said it was normal to lose sensation in my extremities and to be careful navigating stairs because my toes wouldn't be able to sense where the next step was.

He asked me if I played any musical instruments and I said I played the flute and the keyboard. He told me to learn the guitar. I wanted to know why and he said that new players often complained of sore fingers, and that if I was going to learn guitar anytime, I should do it when I couldn't feel my hands hurting.

Dr. Harris finished joking about my musical capabilities and then asked my mother to leave the room so he could talk to me alone. I wasn't in such a great mood and I didn't want to talk to him when he asked me if my hair was falling out yet.

I think the most mature thing I did ever since I was diagnosed was bursting into tears right then. I finally gave in to my situation and cried about something important to every girl; about something that I had kept brushing away up to that point.

I got over it quickly and Dr. Harris was really nice about it and said he dealt with girls crying all the time, so I shouldn't feel too bad about it.

He was totally the nicest man in the world.

It was funny, but I never really had time to cry. Neither did my mother or father or anyone else in my immediate circle of family and friends. I think people thought we were the most hard-hearted people in the world, but really, we were too busy to cry.

The whole Hodgkin's thing was such a whirlwind. There was so much going on at once that we were too overwhelmed to stop and have a good sob. The days were so full, packed with appointments and checkups and blood counts, who could think about how we felt?

Of course, there were times when we had a little free time to think and worry, and that's when we used to break down. But in general, even though I've never asked, I think most people don't cry going through all of it. It's just a distraction.

I needed that cry with Dr. Harris about my hair, and then I was good to go for another while. For now it was just good enough to go home.

We filled up on gas ($1.56 per gallon), and then my mother offered to take me to the mall for smaller clothing on the way home from Hackensack, but I asked her if it was okay to just go straight home.

She said chemo had addled my mind, and that I would one day regret the time I turned down a shopping trip for a whole new wardrobe. And as a tribute to my mother and to all moms out there, I must put it into print for eternity: Mother is always right!

Miss Riegler welcomed me home that night by coming over to help me catch up in Math. She made the tutoring session more enjoyable by bringing over some ice cream and milk-shakes. I had no appetite, but my siblings made quick work of them.

When Miss Riegler had gotten me up to where I was supposed to be in Math, and my sisters and brothers were all in bed, I begged my mother to shave off my hair. She didn't want to. I had to take another shower and watch my hair make a mess on the floor of the tub. It was sickening.

I would have cried all night, but I was too tired.

Tuesday, December 02, 2003

From Boyish to Baldiε

Tuesday was a really full day.

The first big thing that happened was that my first cousin Leiba Levy told us she was getting engaged that night. Well, she didn't tell us, Chavy did. Chavy and Leiba were the same age and were pretty close as cousins, friends, classmates, and any other imaginable way they could think of being together while excluding me.

Even though Chavy called to brag to me that she knew before anyone else that Leiba was getting engaged and to whom, I didn't let her annoy me too much, because I was still excited for my cousin. It was a *simchah* no matter when I found out about it.

As soon as things began to settle and I started to worry about wearing a sheitel to Leiba's engagement, my cousin Chaya Rubinstein called and asked if I wanted company for lunch that day. I told her I didn't mind the visit, but that I didn't have much of an appetite. She said she was coming anyway.

I refused to get dressed, and I ate lunch with Chaya still in my pajamas and robe. Then, as I was walking her to the door, I got two more visitors, Morah Templer and Mrs. Kohn. It was kind of embarrassing.

I could have kicked myself for going to the door in my p.j.'s again. Last time I did that Miss Riegler greeted me, and this time I was no less mortified.

After that was done, my Uncle Yitzchok Meir came over to bring me a gift. He said he had heard what Dr. Harris said about the numb fingers, and he wanted to help me out. As soon as he said that, my Aunt Suri came in, dragging a huge box with a big blue bow on top.

It was a Yamaha acoustic guitar. I called it my new best friend.

My new best friend spent the rest of the evening slung over my back. In my nightclothes and messy hair, my father said I looked like a '60s-style hippy. It was funny.

Another funny thing was my sister Nechama's reaction when I gave her a handful of hair and then walked away. When she realized I was halfway across the room and that a hank of my hair was still in her hand, the look on her face was priceless.

My father was about to tell me off for scaring her when she came running over to me and begged me to do it again. My baby brother Yitzy kept bouncing his blonde curls yelling "Uh-gen! Uhgen!" as Nechama ran around with clumps of my hair in her hands. It was kind of funny even if it was a little disgusting.

When the little ones were in bed, I took care of the last important thing for the day. I climbed onto the bathroom sink and found my father's shaver on the top shelf of his vanity. I brought it into the kitchen and told my brothers to make me an *upsherin*.

They were so excited to take revenge on the big sister who helped cut their *peyos*, and they couldn't wait to give it right back to me.

Faigy took pictures while my mother frantically phoned Chavy to get her to try and convince me to keep my hair for as long as I could. By the time my big sister understood that I was actually cutting my hair and started getting as hysterical as my mother, my hair was in a pile on the floor.

The pictures Faigy took looked like we were having a big party, and we were, but it was still a little scary to see all my hair in a mess under my feet. It was a relief later to be able to shower without my hair falling out, but my head was awfully itchy with tiny little bits of hair still stuck all over.

I stood under the showerhead and rubbed my head hard, trying to get every last piece of itchy hair off me. It was weird to feel my head so round with no hair to run my hand through.

I poured shampoo into my hands and then remembered that I had no use for that anymore. I should have felt really down about that, but all I remember thinking was that my parents were going to save a lot of money on the expensive hair products I used to use.

After the shower I got the first real glimpse of my bald head. It was very frightening. I looked very different without my hair. My eyes were huge and my nose took over my whole face. My forehead didn't end with a hairline; it just went on and on.

This time I wasn't tired enough to fall asleep without a good cry, so cry I did, but only when no one was looking.

WEdNESday, DECEmbEr 03, 2003

REst of thE WEEk Off ChEmo

*M*iss Riegler was over bright and early to help me with some math concepts I was having a hard time with. She left when Devoiry came to have lunch with me.

It was funny when Devoiry walked in to see me and our teacher eating licorice and learning log arithmetic together. Miss Riegler pretended to be all strict and asked Devoiry if she had permission to be out of school for lunch. Devoiry said she promised to be back in time for Math if Miss Riegler didn't tell anyone she snuck out.

Miss Riegler had to laugh when I started giggling. Devoiry laughed too; I think she was more relieved than entertained.

Pinny came home early from yeshiva and crossed paths with Devoiry as she was leaving. He said he left school with a headache, but he played with his GameBoy the rest of the day. When my mother got home from work and asked him what he was thinking, he said he didn't think it was fair that only I got to be sick. He also wanted his chance to be in a Hatzoloh truck and to get nice presents and to stay home from school.

Even though I thought he was crazy, I understood him fully.

I went to bed that night feeling very guilty.

Motza'ei Shabbos, December 06, 2003

Strawberries and Dreams and Eating Jellybeans

*M*y Neupogen shots were getting excruciatingly painful, so we went to take a blood count the next morning to see if I still needed the shots. It was a pain to get the blood work done in a regular lab as opposed to the lab in Hackensack that had results within the hour and with smiling nurses instead of bored technicians who hadn't even passed their citizenship exams yet.

After all that, I got my sheitel fitted to my newly bald head and then went to replace my too-big wardrobe with a bunch of new skirts.

Running around town after a round of chemo felt like using a cell phone when the battery was half dead. It was like I was pushing myself to see how far I could go before my battery ran empty.

When I finally made it home, I left all the bags on the floor of my room and fell asleep on Faigy's bottom bunk.

Miss Riegler woke me up that evening with milkshakes in four flavors hoping I'd eat at least one of them. I didn't have much of a preference due to my lack of appetite, so I let Faigy and Ruchie have one each and then Miss Riegler picked one and I was left with the strawberry shake. I wasn't hungry for it, but it was still yummy.

The first snowstorm of the school year hit us that Friday and to my luck it was the same day I had an appointment to pick up that sheitel from Clyde. Clyde's place was at least a half-hour's drive from my home in normal weather and we had to do it in the blinding snow. It took us almost two hours to make the trip.

On the way there my mother and I were listening to a speech by Rabbi Orlofsky. He was talking about suffering, but it was the funniest speech I ever heard. We almost didn't get out of the car for our appointment because we wanted to finish the tape. Rabbi Orlofsky deserves a huge thank-you for making me laugh on even my worst days of chemo.

While I was waiting for my sheitel to be finished, a woman waiting there complimented my wig on how natural it looked. I was thrilled. She told me *mazal tov* on my wedding and I blushed and told her that I wasn't married.

She asked me what I meant and to my mother's horror I told the flustered woman that I was a cancer patient, and that I was sixteen and much too young to be married.

After I said it I felt really bad because the lady looked so sorry for asking.

People didn't expect my answers. I didn't mind the questions, but I always felt bad when they looked like they wanted to kick themselves after I opened my mouth.

Miri trudged through the snow together with Ayala after the meal that night to come and visit me. Ayala was staying over at Miri's for Shabbos and she was dying to see me in my new bald look. My neighbor Esty also came over and joined us all in a discussion of how natural my wig looked — and in eating my family out of their nosh closet.

All Played Out

At my cousin Leiba's engagement party Sunday night, many people thought my sheitel was my real hair. One of my younger cousins gave it a little tug to see if it would move. It was a good thing I kicked her before she gave the entire hall a chance to see their reflections in my shiny scalp.

I didn't think I looked all that good in the sheitel yet. I wasn't used to wearing it, and it looked and felt heavy around my pale face. I didn't feel comfortable accepting compliments from people I was sure were lying just to make me feel better.

After a long night out, when Faigy was putting five-year-old Shmully to bed, he told her that he was sad. He said he felt like he had no Mommy or Tatty anymore because they were always so busy with me.

If that's not a guilt trip, I don't know what is. The poor kid wasn't even jealous of my presents. All he wanted were his parents back.

I went to school on Monday, just for the attention.

It was a lot of fun to sit in class with a cap covering my sheitel and not get told to take it off. I think it set a record in my school. The teachers all wanted to talk to me, so I spent a good amount of time in the faculty lounge discovering how much I was really loved by all my educators. They got busy comparing their wigs to mine and of course mine was nicer than all of theirs.

I said something funny and that caused one teacher to say that it was a shame that they had to give away my part in the school play because I couldn't be there. I asked her what she meant, and she said that I was supposed to play a big part in the production that year but that they found someone else to take over because I was sick.

I really felt sick hearing that.

Miss Riegler saved the day for me by saying that I was going to be late for Math and we walked to class together.

Right before I walked in, some classmates snatched my cap off my head, saying that my sheitel was stunning and there was no reason to cover it with a cap. They refused to give it back and I was ready to call it quits on my whole day in school.

When Miss Riegler saw some girls trying to hide my cap in a locker, she made them give it back to me. She said that how I felt was not up to me but at least my hat was, and that it wasn't their business to help me get used to my new look.

There was a girl in my class with whom I had become friendly even before I was diagnosed. Her name was Pessie Miller and she was in the same situation as I was. We both had no good friends in our new class. Our school mixed the classes every year and we both got stuck in a class full of cliques without any group to call our own. We were very different on the outside, but sitting together during enough lunch periods showed us that we were pretty much the same, no matter how different we thought or pretended to be.

Pessie called me that night to tell me how glad she was to see me in school and how much she missed sitting with me at lunch. I liked talking to her. I didn't know her for all that long, but from the time we first sat together eating three-day-old bagels at lunch, we got along really well.

She told me that she was really sorry that some girls took off my cap that day. She said that a teacher in the school had asked them to do it. The teacher wanted the girls to tell me how good I looked without the cap and encourage me to wear the sheitel without it.

When I hung up, I got really angry. I was angry at the people who thought they could tell me how to live and what to do and why. It was as if everyone was an authority on Hodgkin's. I was angry at getting sick in general and at having to miss out on the play I had been waiting to star in since I was four years old. Ever since I was tall enough to look at myself in the mirror, I had been practicing for that lead role. I couldn't wait to get to high school and star in the play. And I finally made it there.

It's amazing how many years of dreams can be washed away in one moment. Cancer never bothered me as much as it did that night. I hadn't felt I was missing out on anything important in life until that moment. But that night I knew I was. I was missing out on what that little girl waving to the mirror always wanted; a chance to shine.

I'm by nature not a crier. Just missing out on the play made me upset, but finding out later that a girl I couldn't stand got a lead role made me want to bawl. This girl wasn't even supposed to be in the play; she had been banned because of her rotten behavior. I don't know what changed when I wasn't around to see it, but I did know that she wasn't getting punished, and instead she was smiling and waving to the audience in my spot.

Years later, whenever I think of the worst part of having cancer, it always comes back to the play. I never regretted the time I was sick. I learned and gained so much from it that it was all sort of worth it. The only thing I will never feel was an even trade was the play. For a sixteen-year-old girl, for anyone really, giving up a childhood dream is something not easily forgotten.

Tuesday, December 09, 2003

Chemo, Round Two

I started chemo again feeling nauseous just by dreading it. The nausea I felt was all psychological, but it wouldn't go away.

I sat in an armchair in one of the examining rooms and refused to let anyone touch my port site to hook me up to the chemo. I was pretty miserable thinking about how sick I was going to feel in a few hours.

The nurses gave me some Ativan to make me sleepy and in a couple of minutes I was calm enough to let them access my port without the risk of being injured on the job.

This time around, the infusion room actually had some kids my age to talk to. There were Cheryl and Melinda, who were both high school students doing their first round of chemo. Our mothers were getting to know each other as we were all playing Nintendo. Cheryl's mother asked my mother how she homeschooled her son. I stopped blowing up an alien on screen long enough to tell her that I was a girl.

Later in the day, when I was given the Bleomycin part of the chemo, I started coughing really badly. Dr. Harris had to come and check it out and they gave me Benadryl. From then on I always took Benadryl at the same time as the Bleomycin. It seemed I was a little allergic to it.

Sue, the child-life specialist at Hackensack, came into the infusion room with a huge roll of paper and spread it onto the floor. She had us all get down and write on it all the things we didn't like about being sick. I wrote about the play and that I hated using the hat. I said that I hated how the Bleomycin made me cough and how much I despised Cytoxin. Losing my hair and feeling sick came right after that.

Between all the kids in the infusion room, we filled that huge poster really fast.

After that came the fun part. We all got empty syringes and bowls of paint and we were told to fill the syringes and squirt the paint all over the paper. It was so much fun. After we used up all the paint, we glued the syringes onto the paper.

I was given the honor of naming it, and I named it "Mess-head," because chemo made our lives a mess.

After chemo my mother didn't want to take me all the way home and then drag me back the next day when I was feeling so ill, so we stayed in a nearby Hilton.

It wasn't a great experience. I would have been a lot happier in my own bed. I was just falling asleep when the home health-care service came to access my port again. Dr. Harris wanted me to be on hydration in the hope that it would help minimize the effects I felt the last time around. The visiting nurse gave me a black backpack with an IV bag and monitor inside and showed my mother how to use it and how to change bags as needed.

I was so miserable all night. I couldn't sleep because I was up every ten minutes to use the bathroom. I was still dizzy and sick, and after a while I just got my pillow and slept curled on the floor near the toilet. It was more convenient that way.

As soon as I fell asleep for the fifth time, my backpack started beeping shrilly. The batteries died every nine hours or so, and I had to keep changing them. My Rav said that if I had to, I was allowed to change the batteries on Shabbos, too.

My dear hydration loved to beep on random occasions. It would beep when it was almost empty, when the batteries were dead, when the bag wasn't upright, and whenever I was just about to go to sleep.

The only fun part about the hydration was getting to wear it to school sometimes and asking people to help me with my bag. When they would ask what the wires were sticking out of it, I would explain that they were hooked up to my chest and giving me fluids. Then I would enjoy watching their faces as they tried to restrain themselves from dropping my bag and running away.

Thursday, December 11, 2003

But I'm Jewish!

*B*ecause Wednesday's chemo was so short, I got to go shopping on the way home from Hackensack. I got a funny book full of trivia and a hairdryer for the hair I didn't have.

We came home to find that a package had come for Faigy from that pen company we had bought the Bop-It pen from. My mother had written a letter to them about how Faigy got the pen as a gift for helping out while her sister was getting treatments, and was so disappointed when it broke.

The company sent her a nice letter telling her that they admired her and the package had about four pens in it. There was a "Bop-It" pen, a pen that had a "Monopoly" game on it, another one with "Operation," and still another with "Sorry!"

My mother called Faigy at school to tell her, and Faigy even asked if she could come home early to see them. My mother told her not to push it. She had enough with one daughter playing hooky all the time.

Miss Riegler came to visit that night, and made my day, even though I didn't understand a bit of the math she taught me. My father was noticing how often she came over and started asking me a bunch of questions about her. He wanted to know why a girl like her was still single, and I told him she just hadn't found someone special enough for her.

He was so surprised to hear that she had diabetes. She was so energetic and always looked amazing; it was hard to believe that someone like her wore a metal tag around her neck with her emergency medical information.

I was not exactly happy to mix into my teacher's personal life, but my father said he was going to get to work on getting her married off. I left him alone with his list of eligible boys, and went to watch my siblings eat the supper I had no appetite to taste.

Because it was December, the local organizations in Hackensack were sending their people around to hand out presents to the kids in the hospital. A big fat Santa from the Hackensack Fire Department came to visit me during my infusion on Thursday. He gave Cheryl an MP3 player and then came over to where I was sitting. He started to hand me an MP3 player of my own, but I blushed and said that I was Jewish.

He pulled at his beard, winked, and asked me in Yiddish if I had been a good girl that year. I was shocked and laughed so hard, I almost yanked out my IV line.

Motza'ei Shabbos, December 13, 2003

More Guilt

Friday night Faigy acted really mean to me. She walked out during our *seudah* and said she was going to sleep over at Chavy's house, where she didn't have to do all of my chores. Shabbos morning she told me that she hated me more than anything else in the world and that she didn't care if I never got better because I was ruining her life.

I knew I was ruining her life. She didn't need to tell me that. The poor kid was home babysitting and cooking suppers while I was getting all the attention.

Without telling her, I asked my parents to think about registering her for a really good summer camp that year. They hadn't even begun thinking about the kids' summer plans because they were so busy with me. I thought Faigy deserved something special and I knew she was dying to go to this camp. My parents promised to look into it. But I still felt guilty.

Motzaei Shabbos Faigy and I had a screaming match in the kitchen and we would have pulled each other's hair out except for the fact that I didn't have any.

Then my mother told us to stop fighting and to get dressed and she took us out to the Chai Lifeline Auction where everyone just stared at my sheitel and green complexion.

What a week.

Sunday, DECEMBER 14, 2003

Parties and Poems

Sunday night Chai Lifeline made a huge Chanukah party for all their patients and families. There were a bunch of Jewish singers there and I spent the whole night trying to get all their autographs. I sent my brothers to go and get them because I was too shy to take care of it myself.

It was kind of awkward there. Even though I didn't mind it, I sort of had the feeling that everyone was looking at everyone else trying to determine who the sick child in each family was.

I did enjoy meeting lots of new people who were in the same situation as I was and who understood me more than other people who never experienced cancer did. I met lots of girls my age who were convincing me to go to Camp Simcha that summer. It sounded so exciting, but I was still so deep into my chemo cycles, that I couldn't think past my next session on Tuesday, much less about camp that summer.

Even before the summer Chai Lifeline was organizing a trip to Florida for their patients. They planned to take us all to Disneyworld in January, and I was really excited to go.

Faigy made friends with some Chai Lifeline "sibs." Sibs were the family members of the sick children. Faigy was a sib and she liked meeting other kids who knew what she was going through.

I saw a girl that night who looked as awkward as I did. She wasn't wearing a sheitel, as far as I could tell, but she was really thin and pale and her parents hung around her almost in the same way my father was keeping an eye on me. I got to talk to her a little during the performances when we sat near each other.

Her name was Michal and she was a year older than me. I wanted to know where she was taking chemo and she got upset at me and said she wasn't sick. I felt kind of stupid.

I think Michal saw that I felt bad, and she explained that her father was a doctor, so they got to go to the party each year. She said that she hated coming because it made her scared to see all the sick people.

I guess I had chemo on the brain. I decided I saw sick kids everywhere. It was so sad to see how many sick people there were in just my community. I was surprised at some of the people I met there too. Lots of people kept their illness a secret and I would have never known they were sick if I hadn't met them at the party.

As we were leaving, we got a huge box full of gifts for the entire family. It was very nice until the kids ripped the entire thing apart and fought over who got what all night.

Pinny claimed that I didn't deserve anything because my

Yiddish-speaking Santa Claus already took care of my gifts. I was too exhausted to point out to him that everything I got in the hospital I had already divided up between my brothers. I didn't get anything from the Chai Lifeline box that night.

I was tired and a little depressed that night, but instead of going to bed, I sat at the computer while talking to Miss Riegler on the phone. She was also having a hard time that night. Her parents had been pursuing a promising *shidduch* for a while, but the boy's family called that night to say that they weren't interested. They thought Miss Riegler was a great person, but they didn't want to get involved with someone who was not "perfect."

In other words, Miss Riegler was "damaged goods."

As we were talking, I took something that Miss Riegler said, and put it to rhyme. It came out pretty good for someone who was tired and sick when writing it.

I stuck it into my journal that night as part of my diary. I didn't even show it to my mother until a while later. Somehow people got copies and I've seen it floating around. I don't mind. I wrote it when I needed to hear something like that, and if it makes others feel as good as it made me feel, then that's what it was for.

> *He's Holding My Hand*
> *Sometimes things, they just go wrong,*
> *And there's no logic as far as we can see.*
> *We all react in different ways,*
> *But most of us ask, "Why me?"*
> *But there is logic behind it all,*
> *A reason for our tears.*
> *And the only one Who knows that secret,*
> *Is Hashem, Who really cares.*
> *It's like this mashal I once heard,*
> *That sort of helped me understand,*

Where Hashem is compared to our father,
And we're compared to children in His hands.
You see, when a child is with his father,
He doesn't look if it's okay to cross the street,
He can just close his eyes and take his father's hand,
And then follow in his lead.
Because a child trusts his father implicitly,
He knows he'll never be led astray.
I know that He'll look out for the dangers
    that I might miss,
And then He'll lead the way.
If we follow our Father, Hashem,
He'll lead us on a direct path.
And then we find that our questions may
    be answered,
Before they're even asked.
Of course we all have the option,
Of letting go, and taking our own lead.
Though it's so much easier to rely on a Father
Who takes care of all our needs.
But every father has his secrets,
That is understood.
And some of these things should be kept hidden,
It's all for his child's good.
Yes, every child will sometimes get hurt;
It's just something we can't understand.
But in the end it'll all be okay,
If we keep hold of our Father's hand.
This mashal gave me a bit of knowledge,
That brought tremendous relief.
I now know that it's not about understanding,
But just a matter of belief.

Monday, December 15, 2003

Blurt!

I was taken in to the hospital on Monday because I felt faint. It turned out that my hemoglobin was low and the nurse sent me home, cheerfully assuring me that it would only get lower and that she couldn't wait to see me back for a blood transfusion.

I was jumping for joy.

Later that night, I got a Chanukah present from Miss Riegler. She sent over my all-time favorite board game, "Blurt!" The game is played by one person reading aloud a definition taken from a dictionary while the rest of the players try to blurt out the word being defined before everyone else. It usually ends up very funny when so many people are screaming and trying to say the word that's on the tip of their tongue.

I already owned the game, and Miss Riegler didn't know that no one would play it with me because I always won, but that wasn't the best part of her gift. The cutest thing was the poem she sent along with it.

BLURT!

When you're feeling down and kinda sicky
And life seems like it's very icky,
And you greet visitors halfhearted
And they say things that sound retarded,
Just think of Blurt!
The game where people shout and scream
And don't know what they really mean,
And are busy yelling themselves blue,
Not bothering to listen to you!
It's the game of Blurt!
When the nausea from chemo totally gets you,
And it seems like normal people just forget you,
And when the callers just invade your space,
And you feel like yelling them into place,
Just think of Blurt!
The game where it's about YOU winning
And where the thinking stops right at the beginning,
Like when chesed people come to call,
And don't know what they are doing at all!
It's the game of Blurt!
When people talk without using their brains
And Blurt! out things that sound insane,
Just laugh and try to join the fun,
And then you'll end the game before everyone —
Just think of Blurt!
Where players don't know what cancer is like
And try to do good, though it don't come out right

And I guess you're doing a mitzvah just to let them
And then they finally leave and you can forget them!
It's the game of Blurt!
I know that Blurting is not your speed,
But you need to think that they're in need
They need to feel good about who they are,
And use you to do chesed and maybe get far
Just think of Blurt!
But in the end you come out the winner
(C'mon, chemo makes you sick kids so much thinner!!)
And the other players think they won too,
It's really all up to you!
It's the game of Blurt!

I thought the poem was hysterical. Miss Riegler and I kvetched so much about how people said such inconsiderate things about our situations and this was a cute reminder that they were only trying to do *chesed*. We both agreed that people doing *chesed* who didn't know what they were doing could get on one's nerves, but I guess I was doing more *chesed* by letting them think they were doing *chesed* for me.

The thing with *chesed* is that it's very hard to know where the limits are. I know that everyone just wanted to do something, but often they passed those boundaries. People who weren't close to me would suddenly be calling every night and asking personal questions, and I felt so uncomfortable.

Not everyone did, though. My mother's friend from way back in high school sent her a letter when she heard that I was sick. She wrote that she wanted to help out as much as she could but she felt funny because she and my mother hadn't kept in touch over the years, and she didn't know if my mother wanted her to pop in on our lives.

The letter made a big impression on my mother because it was genuine and was not invading our personal space. Writing a letter meant more than just a phone call because it was something permanent, my mother was able to read it over again and be inspired every time she did. You can imagine that she and her friend became close again in no time.

I think that the whole Blurt! problem and a lot of other annoying parts of *chesed* could be solved by sitting down to write a letter when you really want to help someone. Putting words down on paper really helps set a perspective straight. It's hard to write something that you don't really mean, and looking back at something you wrote shows you what you really feel and what your course of action regarding *chesed* should probably be with that person.

In other do-gooder news, Miss Riegler and I both came to the conclusion that in the *chesed* world there are two types of people: the Nodders and the Strokers. The Nodders are definitely the more pleasant variety to deal with. They are the quiet helpers who nod when you walk into a room, let you know they acknowledge your situation, and do what they need to do in a quiet, non-invasive way.

The Strokers, on the other hand, are the patient's worst nightmare. They are the ones who run over to you as soon as you walk into a room and begin hugging you and stroking your arms, and telling you that all will be well. They talk endlessly about how much *Tehillim* they are saying and that if there's anything you might need, they are always there. The Strokers all seem to have a permanent crease between the eyebrows from where their brows are always furrowed in some sort of sorrowful emotion. If they are the kind of Stroker that can actually end a conversation, it will most likely end off with a hug and even a kiss.

It seemed so twisted yet funny.

Like Blurt!

Tuesday, December 16, 2003

The Faint, the Flu, and the Photo

*B*efore starting chemo Tuesday, the Hackensack Fire Department sent over yet another Santa to visit us kids. This one gave me a set of porcelain dolls. I needed dolls as much as my brother Pinny did, but it was still nice.

Santa then went around posing for pictures with all the children. I told him I was Jewish, he told me he didn't discriminate.

I took the picture.

My father thought it was the funniest thing. I ripped it up after he said he was going to show it to my school.

I got a flu shot that day and it made me sick all night. My parents made me sleep on the floor of their bedroom because they wanted to be near in case something went wrong at night.

But nothing happened that night. They didn't have to worry until the next morning.

Motza'ei Shabbos, December 20, 2003

Sirens, Ambulances, and Emergencies

Wednesday morning I woke up feeling awful. My stomach hurt so much that I couldn't move and it hurt even to breathe. I spent the day in my mother's bed, trying not to cry and trying to sleep at the same time.

The cleaning woman was the only one home with me and she felt bad that I wasn't eating so she brought me a cup of orange juice. I couldn't even sit up to take it from her, much less drink it, but I forced a little bit down to make her happy.

I stayed that way all day until my mother got home from

work. She immediately called the hospital and told them how awful I felt. Ann, the PA there, told my mother that laxatives and Ativan would be a lovely combination considering the way I was feeling, and that if I got any worse, I should be brought to the Emergency Room.

I didn't want to spend more time in the hospital; so instead, I locked myself in the bathroom

It was a bad idea.

As soon as I locked the door I fainted and fell against it. My father managed to unlock the door, but he couldn't open it because I was lying right in front of it.

I have no idea how they got me out in the end, but the next thing I knew there were a bunch of Hatzoloh people taking my pulse and carrying me out to an ambulance so that the entire neighborhood could see.

I was in the Emergency Room for four hours, where they took my blood pressure what felt like forty-five times until it stabilized. I had to go for a stomach x-ray to see why I was in so much pain.

I didn't let anyone near me, and by the time I was installed in a room in the children's ward of the building, the hydration began to work. It turned out that the Vincristine that I was taking as part of chemo was drying me out. My body was dehydrated because of it. Dr. Harris said that from now on he wanted me on hydration all the time.

He might have been a great guy, but I wasn't too happy with him at the moment.

I was so excited about the hydration that I vomited. The first thing I noticed was that I was vomiting pure undigested orange juice. My body was so dry that everything was staying in my body and nothing was being digested. That's why I was in so much pain. Everything I had eaten in the last week or so had turned to rock inside me.

Ouch.

Dr. Harris wasn't on call in the inpatient ward that week, so I had Dr. Roberts instead. He was very nice, and all I wanted to know was why all the doctors there had last names that were also first names. My father wanted to tape my mouth shut, but Dr. Roberts didn't mind me, and he even said that I could go home for Shabbos Chanukah if I promised to report any fevers and keep my mouth covered with a surgical mask against germs.

I was so excited to go home the next morning. I suggested to my grandfather, who'd come to pick me up, that he fill up on gas (by now $1.59 a gallon) before we left, and he said it might be worth it to drive in to New Jersey every time he had to fill up because the price of gas in New York was insane. I didn't care much. I was still only sixteen, nowhere near filling up my own car any time soon.

I didn't have any clothing with me other than those that I had come in and my coat, so when my grandfather drove me home he had to stand guard outside the car door and tell me when the coast was clear so that I could run into the house.

Of course, I ran into the house and the first people I bumped into were a husband and wife who were staying in our guest rooms for Shabbos.

They were a little shocked, but I assured them that I was fine and that even though I was bald, I was still pretty normal.

Another display of my maturiosity.

After Shabbos, my grandfather made a Chanukah party for all the cousins but I couldn't go because I was in isolation. I told my mother to send regards to my Uncles Shimi and David who had both donated blood for me and told everyone to bring me back doughnuts. My father stayed home to babysit me, and I called Miss Riegler over for some company.

Miss Riegler and I played board games and talked and

laughed and made microwave popcorn while my father peeked in every ten minutes to make sure I was still breathing and that my mask was on.

After Miss Riegler had gone home, my father told me that he had a perfect *shidduch* for her. He was divorced, a few years older than she was, working, had a great personality and a good sense of humor and everything else one is supposed to have when in *shidduchim.*

I wasn't listening to him. I told my father that I was not going to set my teacher up with someone and that I didn't feel comfortable doing that and that I didn't know what she was looking for and that it was none of my business.

My father insisted that it was something to consider.

At that moment all my siblings marched in, so that was the end of the conversation.

Sunday, DECEMBER 21, 2003

Second Life Lesson About Pajamas

wo friends called my mother at about nine on Sunday morning to ask if it was okay to come over and visit with me. I was officially in isolation, but my friends couldn't understand that, so I just said it was okay to come over.

I waited all morning for them to come, but they didn't show up. While I was waiting, I began to feel sick and really wanted to take a nap. I should have just called my friends and asked them what was up, or even asked them to come another time, but I felt so bad about being out of the social scene for so long I just waited for them to come.

My friends showed up at three in the afternoon. By that time I was faint and weak and really in need of a nap. I should have told them something but I felt bad because I knew they really wanted to be there for me and they didn't understand what it meant for me to wait up for them all day.

They stayed for three hours and left when my father was ready to light the Chanukah menorah. As they were leaving, one of the girls told me that she was so relieved to have gotten out of the house that day because everyone in her family had the flu.

My parents were livid.

I had just gotten a flu shot and was wearing a mask all day so I was pretty much protected, and I didn't expect my friends to know everything about what it meant for me to be sick, but I did expect some common sense. I thought she should have known better than to come over and spread germs when I had no immune system to speak of.

I wanted to go and nap after we lit the menorah, but my friend Toby called from Lakewood. She always made me laugh and as tired as I was, she was so worth talking to. We spoke very infrequently, but when we did, it was always as if we had just spoken the day before. After just five minutes, she had me feeling so much better about my day.

My father called me into the dining room just as I was making my way upstairs for my long-awaited nap. I stomped back down the stairs in the pajamas and robe I had been wearing all day, and pulled open the door to the room.

Right away I saw that my father wasn't alone. There was another man in the room with him. I thought I was going to cry. I was not up for more visitors, especially some guy I didn't know. I told my father that I was too old to be introduced before I got dressed. My father said I could wrap my blanket around my waist and come in for a minute.

I never win.

I waltzed right in wearing a bright red blanket for a skirt, a hat over my bald head, a mask covering my pale face, and weighing no more than eighty-seven pounds.

Before I even knew who my visitor was, I told him that he was keeping me from taking a nap. He laughed and said it was okay; he didn't need to talk to me for more than five minutes.

My father wasted no time introducing Yossi Spitzer as the man he wanted Miss Riegler to meet.

I had conniptions right then and there. I stomped my foot like a royal queen wearing a red blanket instead of a ball gown. I protested that my father should have warned me that he was coming and I would have at least worn my other blanket.

Yossi assured me that he had seen all of his nieces in blanket gowns before and that I didn't have to worry about that. He said that he came to hear about Miss Riegler and he understood that I was sick and not up to looking decent for visitors.

What a great impression I must have made on the man my father wanted my teacher to marry ....

Actually, I already knew Yossi. He and my father davened together in the same shul every Shabbos. Yossi's father and my father sat at the same table and knew each other from way back. I remembered Yossi as part of the group of boys who threw candies at the girls who came to shul. For Miss Riegler's sake, I hoped he had changed at least a little bit since he was nine.

First off, we established that I was going back to bed in five minutes. Everyone was okay with that. I started counting but I lost track of time after forty-five seconds. We spoke for three full hours.

Yossi wanted to know if Miss Riegler had a first name. It turned out that Miss Riegler's name was a problem; Yossi's mother was also named Mindy. I said that I thought she had a second name so maybe it would be okay, but it didn't really matter.

It didn't take the full five minutes I had promised to see that Yossi was not for Miss Riegler at all. His sense of humor wasn't her speed and the topics we spoke about weren't in Miss Riegler's field of interest either. I told him that he was out of the running about ten minutes in, but he shrugged and laughed and said, "Can't win them all!"

We touched upon the whole school system in conversation and I said something to the effect that I wanted to be a teacher when I grew up, because I wanted to help change the system and make it better for my kids eventually. I had no idea where that came from because I had never wanted to teach before. I guess being sick did something to change the way I thought and felt about things.

Yossi wanted to know how I felt about all my visitors and the outside world from my new perspective. I asked him if he had about three days to listen to me vent.

I complained about the people who viewed cancer as some catchy plague and treated me as if I were inferior to everyone who never had anything troublesome in their lives. I asked him what was wrong with our community that made people like me, older singles, divorcees, children from broken homes, and others who didn't fit the perfect mold of society, into second-class citizens.

Yossi laughed at that and said that he identified with what I was saying because as a divorcé, he was set up with his share of "interesting" girls. He said he hated to break it to me but when I would be closer to *shidduch* age, the *shadchanim* would think I was only suitable to be set up with men who were sick or also viewed as "damaged" by our community.

I was more angry than upset about that. Yossi wasn't telling me anything I didn't know, but I was hurt that just because I was walking around bald for a few months, it meant that one day I would be considered "not good enough" for someone's son.

My father said I couldn't fight the system. If I lived here I was doomed to play by the rules. I told him that it didn't bother me to marry someone who was special and different like I was, what bothered me was that people like us were viewed differently and judged unfairly.

I felt that I was becoming a stronger and better person because of my experience and I imagined that other people in hard situations also grew from them. I was bothered by the idea that one day the news would spread that I was a *kallah* and instead of "mazal tov" the first thing people would say would be, "But she had *cancer*! What was wrong with the boy that he took her?"

Yossi admitted that it was sad, but that *im yirtzah Hashem* I would have the last laugh by marrying happily. Our community gives the impression that they don't expect people like me and Yossi and others considered "damaged" to make it; so when we do, and we do it well, we are the ones who shock everyone and end up winning.

I remarked that I didn't want to marry a "normal" boy anyway, because a boy who hadn't gone through something trying in his life wouldn't be on my level of maturity. My brother-in-law Eli walked in just as I was saying that part about being mature and he and my father laughed and nudged each other.

I was so embarrassed.

Then Chavy walked in and gave me a "look" that said, "Oh please, don't tell me you're still not dressed!"

I was embarrassed further.

I tried to fix it up by saying that I wasn't perfect, but that I thought I wanted to marry someone a little older than me with some life experience.

My father, Eli, Chavy, and Yossi all told me to get a little older first.

It's like it was a crime for me to forget once in a while that I was only sixteen.

Eli piped up and said that he actually had a friend who had Hodgkin's just like I did and that maybe when we both got better, and a little older, we could get married. I snubbed him and said that I would never marry his friend because he was not old enough for me and because he was probably a *shtreimel* kind of person.

Yossi asked me what was wrong with a *shtreimel* and my father told him not to get me started.

I had nothing against men who wore them, but I didn't want one for myself. I didn't go to a chassidishe school and it was not what I had in mind for my future. In fact, I was a little surprised when I saw Yossi with a beard. It took me a second to register the idea that Miss Riegler was probably looking for someone with the whole chassidishe *levush*. It was so out of my frame of mind because it wasn't what I intended for myself.

Yossi pretended to be upset because he wore a *shtreimel* and I said, "And that's why we were setting you up with Miss Riegler, and not with me!" He thought that was funny.

My father became bored when Yossi and I were conversing so nicely without him, so he changed the topic and told Yossi all about the many Santa Clauses I met in the hospital.

When Yossi left my house at 11 p.m., he knew all about David and Louis and Steve. He promised to come and visit another time, but I hoped he'd stay away long enough for me to live down the entire embarrassing conversation ... and the fact that it was all done in a bald head, hospital mask, robe, and a red blanket wrapped around my waist.

After he left, my father exhausted me further by making me take apart and analyze the night and tell him what I thought about Mr. Perfect for Miss Riegler. I told him there was no chance that those two were ever going to go out.

My father tried making me see reason by pointing out how funny and intelligent Yossi was. I put an end to the discussion by saying that if he insisted that I marry a *shtreimel* personality then a younger version of Yossi would do nicely for me, but Miss Riegler was out of the question.

Faigy overheard my comment and started singing that I wanted to marry Yossi Spitzer. She and Chavy began calling me Mrs. Spitzer.

Sisters can be so weird. The guy was older than Miss Riegler, which meant he was much older than me. Because he was already once married, he wore a *shtreimel* every week, and he also had the one surname I swore I would never have. I knew a Mrs. Spitzer in elementary school whom I absolutely abhorred. She was my teacher in second grade and she was so mean. She never let her students go out to use the bathroom during class and she hardly ever let us color our handouts with markers. She never smiled and she used hard words that none of us understood.

I once went to pick up my sister Ruchie from school and passed Mrs. Spitzer in the hallway. I was already in high school but when I passed her she still gave me the same mean look she used to use on me in second grade, and I was ready to run into the corner before she could put me there herself.

The woman was awful. There was no way I was ever going to turn into a Mrs. Spitzer. In a way I was happy Yossi wasn't going to go out with Miss Riegler. I didn't want her to be a Spitzer either.

After throwing a cookie at Faigy and hiding Chavy's car keys on the top of the bathroom vanity, I remembered I was tired and cranky, and I went up to bed.

Finally.

Monday, December 22, 2003

Is Unwanted Chesed Still Chesed?

We woke up bright and early Monday morning so that I could take some tests.

I had already done echocardiograms and electrocardiograms before, but I needed to take more so that the doctors could keep monitoring my heart on chemotherapy.

I went to the clinic, where they stuck my hand but got no blood in return. Instead, I had the pleasure of being stuck again via a finger stick. I hated them worse than regular blood drawing. I would much rather they accessed my port.

The first IV line they put in that didn't yield any blood was just left in my arm so that the CT scan place would be able to use it later.

Oh joy.

I was the girl who fainted regularly at the sight of blood, but here I was, begging them to take the IV out and then stick me again later when they needed to.

In the end, sitting with that IV stuck in my arm wasn't as painful as I thought it would be. They accessed it at the CT scan place for the contrast, and that meant that I tasted helium in my mouth, felt hot all over, and had that general uncomfortable feeling. By the time all the scans were done, I really needed a good nap.

I was doing all the scans because I was just finishing my second round of chemo. I chose to go on the new treatment where I might end up getting four cycles of chemo instead of eight, and that meant that I had to get tested after my second cycle to see how many more cycles I would need. If I was all clean, no tumors anymore, then I only had to take another two rounds of chemo and then maybe get randomized not to have radiation. So my mother and I were running around all day trying to find out what was going on inside my body.

I thought it was so ironic that there were people out there who thought that cancer patients were not worth getting involved with come *shidduchim* time. People assume that cancer patients are going to be ill for life. The truth is, though, that people like me are more up-to-date with everything going on in our bodies than those people who claim they are healthy as an ox and haven't been to the doctor in ten years.

On the way home we got a call that there was one part of the bloodwork that the technician had somehow forgotten to do or misplaced, and would we mind coming back to get it done. By that time we were almost home, and we didn't like the idea of going back for one little tube of blood. My mother made a few frantic phone calls and spoke to Nancy the PA and then Nancy spoke to Dr. Roberts, who was on call that day instead of Dr. Harris, and then she called my mother back to tell her that I could take the blood test locally and then have the lab fax them the results.

We then went back to the Rite Aid pharmacy where I took my original bloodwork before my whole Hodgkin's saga began, and surprisingly, we were able to go right in! I waited in the chair while my mother arranged my insurance, and I watched the tech stick some other people. As I waited, a girl in a school uniform came in and handed the technician a script for some bloodwork she needed done.

She looked around as she was getting her blood taken and when I saw her face I realized that it was Michal, the girl I had met at the Chai Lifeline Chanukah party. She saw me at the same time I saw her and she looked like she was going to cry. I felt bad, so I just gave her a small wave and pretended to read some pamphlet on liver disease.

I finally got my blood taken, and as I walked out of the office, I bumped right into Michal. Michal looked really shy and asked me to please not tell anyone that I saw her there. I assured her she didn't have to worry.

Then Michal started crying and said that she lied to me at the Chanukah party and that she was sick too and her family was keeping it a secret. She didn't want to tell me what kind of cancer she had but she said that her doctor had told her there was almost no chance she was going to survive it, but they were trying everything they could. Her family felt it best to keep the whole thing under wraps so that she could live as normally as possible.

Michal didn't even want to say the word *cancer*. She looked uncomfortable every time I said it. She even told me to shush when she thought I was about to say the word. I couldn't understand her. I found it so much less scary when I was open about it.

Michal and I sat down on some chairs to talk while my mother pretended to need something from the pharmacy. I was so shocked to hear that Michal was actually going to school every day and also taking chemo. She said she would wake up at four in the morning to go to Sloan Kettering, take her doses and then make it back in time for class. She would be up until about midnight every night so that she could study and make up her work.

I asked her why she was making it so hard on herself and she said that she was a normal girl and that she didn't want anyone to treat her like she was sick. She explained that she was in twelfth grade and graduating that year and wanted to have the best senior year she could. She didn't want to look back at her high-school pictures and think, "Oh that was the year I was sick and missed out on all the fun."

She didn't want to wear a sheitel even though she said she lost a lot of hair. I never knew her before I met her at the Chai Lifeline party, so I didn't know what her hair used to be like.

She said she felt stupid because she didn't even know me and she was spilling her secret in some Rite Aid pharmacy, but I told her it was better that way. I wasn't someone who knew her and her friends, so I couldn't spill the beans to anyone that mattered, and I was also sick so I understood her.

She felt a little better after that and I asked her how she coped with sitting in school every day. Michal said it was very hard, but she wanted to do it. She really wanted to live as normally as she could manage.

My mother "happened" to pop back near us just then, and Michal said she had to go. We exchanged numbers and promised to keep in touch. Michal smiled and said she felt much better now and that she was excited to have someone to talk to who really understood.

I felt guilty when she said that part about me really understanding. I didn't think I really did. My type of cancer had a 98% survival rate while Michal was told flat-out that she wasn't going to make it.

Michal asked me if I was taking chemo and I rolled my eyes and pointed to my bald head. "Good," she said, "so you *do* understand me. Don't worry about survival rates, miracles can happen; do I look like I'm planning to die any time soon?"

"But I'll be done chemo way before you will be," I protested.

"So? In the meantime we are both doing the same thing; same chemo, same bloodwork, same nausea, same horrible time. We can understand each other no matter how different our outcomes may one day be."

I found Michal to be an amazing person. She just took things in stride with such a great attitude. And people think *we* need the *chizuk*!

On the way home with my mother, I burst into tears. I told my mother that Michal said her cancer wasn't definitely curable, and I didn't know how she was so normal even though she wasn't sure she was going to make it. It hurt me so much that she was keeping it a secret, because I thought she was just making it harder for herself to cope and that if people knew she could get so much more help and support.

My mother explained that every person has her own way of doing things, and that Michal and her family had to do what they thought best for them. The fact that Michal chose to confide in me meant that she was asking for my support, and I should definitely be there for her.

I was left with a lot to think about.

Back to my much desired nap; it was not to be. I had some visitors come over without calling first and that meant that as tired as I was, I had to entertain them until we lit the menorah.

Right after that we had to run to a Chanukah party. I was still in isolation so I wasn't really allowed to go, but the host of the party promised that it would be a very small get-together and that it would be totally fine.

I don't know about you, but a party consisting of about eighty people isn't a small get-together in my opinion and it definitely isn't "totally fine" for a kid in isolation.

The party was really nice and of course I embarrassed myself when my cell phone rang to the tune of "Yankee Doodle" while somebody was giving a *d'var Torah*.

Somebody at the party bought me a few of Rabbi Orlofsky's tapes, and my mother said she couldn't wait until I started chemo again so that we could listen to them in the car on the way to the hospital. We always saved his tapes for the car rides back and forth; it was when we needed them most.

I gained so much wisdom from his lectures. I finally learned what pestilence meant on his tape, "Why Be Jewish?" My mother and I laughed so hard during that one that we had to get off the highway to regain our composure, because my mother kept losing control of the steering wheel.

I know, I know, we have a warped sense of what is normal.

The Chanukah party dragged on until really late that night, and I was tired and in isolation to begin with. I got a little cranky toward the end, and begged my father to take me home so that I could go to bed, as I had been dying to do for the last seven hours.

When I finally got home I was too tired to climb upstairs to bed, so I stayed in the kitchen complaining about the people who think they are doing *chesed* but are really just a pain in the neck.

This had nothing to do with anyone bothering me; this had to do with me wanting to kvetch.

I complained to my mother that some of my friends thought they were doing *chesed*, but who were they doing it for? It wasn't for me, because to me it was all a bother. I wondered if their unwanted *chesed* counted as a mitzvah even when it achieved the opposite of the desired effect and made me feel worse.

I decided that some people do *chesed* just to make themselves feel good about doing a mitzvah. I thought it might be a good idea to set my voicemail to say, "By calling my number you have just completed your *chesed* for the day! Thank you so much for doing it with me! Don't bother leaving a message, because I won't listen to it anyway, but have a great day!"

My father thought it was a good laugh. My mother thought it was snobbish. I thought it was brilliant.

I begged my father to take me back to Hackensack that night, because my house was a noisy mess with all the kids fighting over Chanukah presents and whatnot. He wanted to know why I thought sleeping in the hospital would be better.

I told him it was because in Hackensack they only woke me up every four hours to give me a sleeping pill and then they left me in peace. My father went and repeated it to the friend he was talking to on the phone.

I called Miss Riegler to vent to her about how horrible it was to be sick and how annoying it was to have a father who liked to embarrass me in front of people I didn't know. Miss Riegler told me all fathers were the same, and that he didn't mean it that way, and that he really loved me. She was getting on my nerves, so I hung up on her, too.

As tired as I was, I still took a sleeping pill before going to bed. I just couldn't wait to fall asleep.

Tuesday, December 23, 2003

Meet My Siblings

ackensack is the best hospital ever. There's this one person there, Judy, who takes care of anything and everything that has nothing to do with being sick. She arranges all the trips and fun stuff for the patients. Every year she arranges the most amazing Chanukah party ever. The party is for all the Jewish patients and their families. There's always lots of food, tons of games, and a really cool performance.

My family was so excited to go, and all my siblings decided to get dressed in matching rugby shirts for the occasion. Even my mother and Chavy wore them. Eli and my father both wore rugby shawls. We looked a little ridiculous, but it was fun.

We were thirteen people all dressed in blue and grey stripes, and I can imagine what a sight we must have been. We probably made everyone around us dizzy.

Someone made an observation to my mother that the shirt she was wearing was so popular; it seemed like everyone at the party was wearing them. My mother smiled and told her, "Yeah, those are all my kids."

The woman was speechless for a minute, and then said, "No, you don't get it, there are like twenty people here wearing that exact shirt!"

My mother grinned and said again, "No, it's *you* who doesn't get it. Those are all *my* kids!"

My father overheard the exchange and piped up jokingly, "And we left the three youngest at home."

I think the woman fainted before he had a chance to tell her he was joking.

Nancy, one of the PA's in Hackensack, passed Zevy and Pinny playing killer tag in the hallways. She told them to be careful, otherwise they could get hurt, and Pinny said, "Who cares? We're in a hospital anyway!"

Nancy decided those two little guys had to be my brothers.

The food was so delicious. They had pizza and doughnuts and a million types of junk food and bagels and a bunch of other things that made my mouth water and my stomach grumble.

I couldn't eat too much because it was the time in my chemo cycle where the Vincristine was kicking in. I kept getting visits from David in my tummy and he also started messing with my head. I told my parents that I couldn't eat because in my head I knew that I had two vegetable turnovers, three pizzas, two-and-a-half doughnuts, and eight rice cakes in my intestines.

Okay, eeew.

Ayala Klein was in Hackensack for the party with her whole family, and I sat near her most of the time. She introduced me to some other people she had gotten to know there over the years of coming back for her brother's checkups and yearly Chanukah parties.

As the day went on, I felt worse and worse, and I was in a whole lot of pain because of my stomach. I begged my parents to take me home, or better yet, leave me in the hospital before Hatzoloh had to take me in again.

But the party ended soon enough, and then as we were leaving, Nechy Berger and her family gave me a beautiful leather-and-silver *Tehillim*. It was so nice of them and really moved me. This is the kind of *chesed* people appreciate; a quiet reminder that there are people out there who care for you. The people who barge into your life aren't the ones who are appreciated, but the ones who make their presence known with a card, a letter, a small gift, or even a short phone call are the ones that make all the difference.

As we were leaving, each family was given a box full of presents for everyone in the family. Of course my siblings started fighting over who got what and I didn't get anything. I didn't care about that because my room already looked like Toys 'Я' Us anyway. It's not like I needed anything, but what bothered me a little was that my siblings didn't think I deserved any of the presents because I already had so much and because I got all the attention from my parents these days.

I knew that they were right, but didn't they have any clue that being sick was no picnic?

While I was sprawled out on the couch later that evening, someone came over to drop something off for my father and he asked my father if I had the flu, because I didn't look so well.

My father looked at him and said, "Uh ... no .... She actually got the flu shot already, so she's set, she's just a little under the weather now with cancer."

The look on the man's face was priceless. Now I was just waiting for him to send me a present.

Wednesday, December 24, 2003

Tired, Moody, and Stuck in Traffic

I was terribly nauseous the next morning when my mother drove me down to Hackensack for more scans. She gave me a Phenergen tablet to ease my nausea, but it made me incredibly sleepy.

The tech at the PT scan place was dressed as if he were expecting a nuclear bomb to fall any second. He wore protective goggles, gloves, and an extra lab coat. He pulled a vial out of an isolated container that had three locks on the top of it. The vial was as thick as my arm and made of heavy metal and the tech had to inject that into my arm.

The tech noticed me staring at it and he assured me that while the stuff inside the vial was radioactive, it was totally safe. I wanted to know why he was all in safety gear then.

He ignored me.

I had to wait an hour for the actual scan and I fell asleep waiting. My mother left me with my Aunt Carla and my Uncle Sol so that she could go back to work. I wasn't too happy about being left alone in the hospital when I was so sleepy, but I had no choice. I couldn't keep my mother from going to work every day. I already felt so guilty making her come to Hackensack with me all the time.

As soon as I got into the machine, I fell into the deepest sleep I'd had in ages. I didn't want to get off the table for my next test, the Pulmonary Function Test.

Of course we got lost finding the next scan. My aunt went over to some resident in the hallway to ask him for directions and he said he'd take us there. I asked him why he was being so nice to us and walking us halfway across the campus when he could have just given us directions, and he said that it was part of Hackensack's patient-care policy.

He said that when people started working in an office or clinic in Hackensack, they were given a handbook on how to treat patients. It told them that they had to be honest about the wait-time for a patient, and they had to take people where they needed to go.

As tired as I was, I marveled at the difference between Hackensack and Manhattan. The doctors might be just as good in either place, but the service out of town — whoa. That was amazing.

Even with help, it took a year-and-a half to find the office for the PFT. I had a hard time walking because I was so tired. I just wanted to cry. I was way too zonked to start puffing into tubes like they wanted me to do at the test.

The women doing the tests with me was very talkative and she kept asking me if I had a date to take me to the junior prom at my school. I then had to explain to her that I went to a religious all-girls' school and that we didn't have proms. She felt so sorry for me.

She wanted to know how I handled being in a different school than my boyfriend.

I told her it was fine.

Then I shocked the woman by performing so well in my breathing tests that my results came out exactly the same as they were before I even started chemo. It was the same down to the last decimal.

I guess that's where all the *Tehillim* being said had an effect.

I still had to go to the clinic for a complete blood count and the results came out great! I was allowed to stop my GCSF shot that night! I was so excited to stop taking them.

As I was waiting for a Chai Lifeline volunteer to take me home, one of the nurses gave me a gift. It was a board game called "The Game of Life."

Finally, the Chai Lifeline driver showed up, and then things started going wrong. The driver didn't speak English fluently, and he didn't know the way to where I lived. I was too tired to focus on my Yiddish to direct him, so I had him talk on the cell phone to my father, who had to get him home through all the holiday traffic. The usual forty-five-minute ride took two hours.

I tried calling Michal to complain, but she had her own complaining to do that day. Her best friend from the hospital had gone into a coma the night before. This girl was not raised frum but started learning more about *Yiddishkeit* when she became sick. Michal spoke about Shira like she was the most special person in the whole world.

It was hard to hear everything Michal was saying because she started to cry and couldn't stop. That made me start crying, too. I was crying for Michal and for her friend and for me, stuck in traffic and dead tired.

It made me so miserable thinking of the reality of our situation. For me, Hodgkin's was something I took in stride, something I did day to day. Michal and her friend were the same way. None of us expected this harsher side, even though it was always there under the surface. I never knew Michal's friend, but hearing that someone so close to her was close to dying was so scary.

I have no recollection of what I told Michal then and of the rest of the conversation because I was so drugged up. I literally kept pinching myself to stay awake, but the Phenergen was so strong that it was still making me sleepy. Whenever I would suddenly jerk awake, I would have to talk to myself to keep from crying when I would see how much traffic we were stuck in. All I wanted was to get home and crawl into bed.

When I finally staggered through the front door, Faigy made it impossible for me to get any sleep. She was hosting a class Chanukah party and she was yelling nervously at all my brothers who were busy messing up all her hard work.

Annoyed, I got out of bed and told her that I had gotten her something she really needed: a life. I gave her the game I got in the hospital that day and she seemed much happier after that.

Later, the younger kids all went over to neighbors while Faigy had fun with her guests.

The next day, Morah Templer and her daughter came over with a gift for me and a bunch of yummy doughnuts for everyone else. Then my neighbor Esty came over to have me listen to a speech she gave her school about *Perek Shirah*. She was the *chesed* head in her school and she gave out small *Perek*

Shirah pamphlets with my Jewish name put on the cover. I thought it was such a nice thing.

I needed a cry later so I called Miss Riegler. She was dialing me as I called her. She also needed to vent. She was over at a class Chanukah party reunion, and she and two other girls were the only ones not married yet. She felt so out of place and left early.

We spoke for a while and I think we both ended up crying a little and then laughing about it. Having cancer made me so moody!

Halfway Point!

E rev Shabbos my personal phone line rang. It was Dr.
Harris himself, calling to speak to me about the results
of my scans. He said that he was calling to tell me
mazal tov because the scans were beautiful and that meant
I would need only two more rounds of chemo instead of the
usual four.

I thought my doctor was awesome for calling to tell me the
news personally. He made all his patients feel like he came to
work each morning just for them.

Say it with me: he's such a mentch.

My family was so excited. I knew this was really only the
halfway point, but it seemed so much shorter now that I saw
the end of the treatments approaching.

I called Michal to tell her the good news, and she was genuinely happy for me. She told me that over the last week she had some scans done and they showed some improvement. I was happy to hear that too, but it made me sad to think that Michal had no idea when her halfway point might be. She was being given chemo just to see if it even made a difference to her situation, and then when it started working, they were going to give her a more definite regimen.

Michal told me not to feel bad for her or else she was going to stop talking to me. I quickly assured her that I had no reason to feel bad for her other than the fact that she didn't get as good presents for Chanukah as I did.

Michal said she forgave me and then told me that she had been in school the day before and the teacher had put a bunch of names on the board to say *Tehillim* for and that mine was one of them. She said it was so strange for her to read the names and realize that she personally knew about half of them from Memorial Sloan Kettering.

That is a weird feeling.

I asked her how her friend was doing and she said she kept going to visit her and tried talking to her, but it was too much. She sounded about to cry talking about it, and said I shouldn't think about it when it was such a happy time for me.

Sunday afternoon I finally got my second sheitel. My Aunt Suri drove me out to where Clyde had her salon and we picked up my new wig. It took forever for Clyde to see us, but I left there with a custom wig that fit perfectly to my bald head. I had to use a special double-sided sticky tape to get it to stay on. I thought it was so strange, but Clyde assured me that when my hair grew in she would sew a comb and clips in for me.

I laughed when she said something about my hair growing in. I was so used to being bald, I couldn't imagine having hair again.

My friend Devoiry's sister got engaged that night and I went to the party, but I didn't wear my new sheitel. I still needed time to get used to it before wearing it outdoors comfortably.

The engagement was beautiful and so was the *kallah,* of course, but I was afraid, because I was still in isolation and I wasn't wearing a mask. My parents weren't too thrilled about that because I had to go in for chemo the next day.

Eventually I left and my mother took me to my friend Malky Gold's house for a belated Chanukah party. Malky was a friend from camp, and she was two years older than me. Everyone at her party was at least two years older than I was, but I had a great time anyhow.

Then my mother picked me up and reminded me that I had a full day of chemo coming up. What a bummer.

Monday, December 29, 2003

I HATE the Energizer Bunny!

r. Harris found it interesting that I was always getting nauseous on the way to the hospital, even before I took any drugs. He thought it might be because of nerves and prescribed Ativan before each day of chemo. After drugging me up on Ativan, we left the house at seven in the morning to start my third round.

It wasn't as bad as it could have been, because I had taken the Ativan before, but I didn't like feeling so disoriented all day. I couldn't focus on anything and spent all day sitting in the infusion room, staring at the ceiling.

Sue Daniels came in later to tell me that the painting we had made the last time with the syringes was entered into an art competition that had a special exhibit created by kids with illnesses. She asked me to write something to be on display near the painting and I did write something, but I can't remember what it was because I was so drugged up. I hope I didn't embarrass myself!

She also read some of my writings and said I should publish them. If I ever do publish anything, I'll have to tell people it was because of her!

I don't remember the rest of the day. I was so sick and drugged up that everything was a blur. When I got home I was too sick to move around on my own, so my father had to carry me up the stairs and he put me in my mother's bed for the night. When I woke up I had no idea why I was there and how I had gotten there. I was so out of it.

I had been sent home with the portable IV. It was so annoying, half the time the batteries would die and the machine would beep incredibly loudly until I dragged myself out of bed and changed the stupid batteries.

NEVER NEVER EVER will I believe another stupid Energizer advertisement. There is NO SUCH THING as the Energizer bunny that just keeps going and going and going and going and going and going. ENERGIZER BATTERIES DIE DIE DIE AND DIE AGAIN JUST LIKE ALL THE OTHER BRANDS!

I feel so much better now.

I texted Michal at two in the morning, just because I had nothing better to do. She texted back that she was spending the night in the hospital and she was lonely. She had fainted in the grocery that morning and had to go in to the hospital overnight to be under observation.

We had a nice conversation where Michal told me in detail (in numerous short and choppy text messages) how her parents got a call that morning from her *mechaneches* because her teachers were worried about how thin she was getting. Her teacher thought she was becoming anorexic and recommended that her parents take her to a nutritionist and a psychologist and go through the works. Michal thought it was so funny.

I thought it was so sad. If Michal were open about her being sick, even if just to the teachers, she would gain their understanding and support instead of being misunderstood by people who really cared about her.

I knew that it wasn't any of my business and that Michal was happy the way she was dealing with her situation, just as I was comfortable with my way. I wanted Michal to have it easy, but from talking to her I could tell that she thought that telling people about being sick was going to make her as miserable as it would make me to keep it a secret.

I think I got myself too confused to focus then because I fell asleep with my cell phone still in my hands.

Tuesday, December 30, 2003

And I HATE Teddy Bears Too!

*T*uesday's chemo was really quick for some reason and we went to the mall afterward. I got a set of science-fiction books that my cousin Chaya told me about, and I was as happy as anything.

The rest of my day was awful. Even with the hydration I still wasn't feeling well.

I had no appetite again and when I decided I wanted a certain milkshake that they only made in one shop across town, my father ran out to get it, but when he got back I didn't want it anymore. He said that I was worse than a woman craving pickles at four in the morning.

Chemo was such a pain.

My neighbor Ruchy Perlstein moved away that night and I was too sick to tell her good bye. I was in a horrid mood.

It didn't help matters when Miss Riegler told me that the teachers in school thought of me as some poor little sick child who needed a lot of cheering up. I know they only meant well, but I was far from being a charity case.

My grade mates all chipped in to buy me a huge white teddy bear that cost something like eighty dollars. It was a pretty bear and all, but it was shedding all over my chair. I was so annoyed. Come on, these were eleventh-grade girls! Did they really think that I needed a teddy bear? If they really wanted to get me something decent, a gift certificate to the local music store would have been just fine. Not as big and plushy as an eighty dollar teddy bear, but more enjoyable and more to the taste of a sixteen-year-old.

Some people just don't think.

And it sounds rude to say this after the girls made the effort to do something nice, but now was when they chose to be nice to me? What about before I got sick? My classmates never really tried to include me when they were in their cliques and I just flitted around from group to group.

There was one particular group in my class that especially enjoyed making my life miserable. They thought I was too much of a fun person to care what they were doing and to notice how they laughed and rolled their eyes behind my back, but unfortunately, I didn't have that hard of a shell.

I say *unfortunately*, because it was unfortunate for me. I would have given anything to be as carefree as they thought I was and maybe miss those snobby remarks and looks. I hurt so much being around those girls, and getting silly teddy bears from them when I knew I meant nothing to them anyway, really bothered me a lot.

I don't know if it was me or them, but teenagers can be cruel. I am older now, married, and have a great life. I am more successful than many of the girls who hurt me in high school, but that pain never went away. No matter how far I have come, I still remember that once upon a time I was an eleventh grader who was used over and over again by some girls who needed an object for their jokes.

Okay, back to what I was saying. I didn't need teddy bears from people who didn't care about me, and I hated the idea that girls were trying to get rid of what may have been their guilty consciences with overpriced presents.

I was on the phone with Miri and she got me to see the ridiculous side of the whole teddy-bear thing. She said we could make tons of money if we set up a photography studio and used the teddy bear in our shots. She offered to come over and try a few shots to see how photogenic my new bear was with her younger brother. We were laughing hysterically in no time.

I may have been overreacting and assuming more than I should have, but that bear hurt so much to look at, and besides, it shed hair all over the place. After a while I just let Yossi Spitzer take it home for his little nephew. I couldn't figure out what it was exactly that I felt about the bear. I guess it was something to the effect that expensive gifts don't help people going through a rough time as much as showing how much you care and meaning the things you say.

One cousin sent my mother a packet of handmade coupons that she had put together for a bunch of different services my mother could redeem. She offered a free supper for the kids, babysitting, and a bunch of other things. My mother never asked for any help, but I saved the coupons and still have them years later. I also saved every letter, card, and helium balloon I got during the time I was sick. The thought and feeling behind each one were what mattered most to me.

I compared the whole present situation to something Rabbi Dovid Orlofsky had said on one of his tapes. He explained that when fans at a baseball game or at a rock concert try to flatter the stars, they aren't doing it to boost the person's ego; they're doing it for themselves. They are hoping that by praising their hero, he will look at them, maybe smile, autograph something, or maybe even shake their hand. They are just hoping to be noticed by the people they idolize.

I know it isn't fair to say this, but I felt that everyone was trying too hard to push things on me, and that not enough of my so-called "fans" cared enough about what I really liked or wanted or felt. It was all about *them*.

I cried forever that night and decided that I was going to quit school.

Yossi was taking the teddy bear to give to his cute nephew, and he overheard me venting. He said it was a good decision to leave because I was too smart for school anyway, and I could come to work for him instead. It sounded like a plan until he admitted that he had the secret motive of hiring someone underage so he could get away cheap on my salary.

I told him he was just as bad as everyone else.

Motza'ei Shabbos,
January 03, 2004

A New Year

Even though my parents didn't want me to, I fought to go to school on January first. They said it was so sad what the chemo was doing to my mind. A few short months before I was the girl who smashed alarm clocks on the first day of class and now after treatments I was slowly losing my mind.

I was going to talk to the principal first to ask if it was okay to just come in and disrupt the class when I had no intention of actually learning anything, but because we were running late, I got to class the same time that my teacher did, and there was no time for permissions.

The school had actually asked my mother to tell them in advance when I planned on coming in, because it turned the school upside-down every time I showed up in a sheitel. I optimistically told myself they wanted notice so they could roll out the red carpet.

I was wearing my IV backpack to school and the girls were all a little awed and afraid of it. It was a great feeling, until it began beeping in class and I got so flustered that it took a while to insert a new bag of hydration.

I was glad that no one had warned the girls that I was coming. They would have been much more reserved and not as normal around me as I would have liked them to be.

A teacher who had sent me out of class the first day of school told me that it was like a *yom tov* when she saw my face among the students in her class. I grinned and wished her a Happy New Year. I think she considered throwing me out of class again, but then reconsidered after remembering that I was bald.

It wasn't the brightest idea to have gone to school when my immune system was in the dumps and I was too shy to wear a mask in public. The girls were all crowding around me the entire day and I was really worried that I would get sick again.

I had already been feeling a little sick the night before, and I had painful blisters on my hands from the Adriamycin chemo I was taking. I also couldn't move around too much or too fast because my stomach was at it again.

Later that night my sister Faigy fainted, and it felt so odd not to be the only sick one in the house. I guess we all got so carried away with my Hodgkin's that it was a small shock to remember that other people get sick too sometimes.

Again, I had a hard time sleeping, so by nine in the morning I was up for hours and had already gotten a lot done. I was bored by 9:30, so I woke up my next-door neighbor, Leah Freund, and made her go shopping with me.

On the way back from shopping, we passed a bunch of little kids who lived on my block. They couldn't stop staring at my bandanna and IV line. I felt kind of stupid.

The day got a little better when my mother made me take a prescription laxative called Lactulose. It tasted like raw eggs and oil, but it worked. I felt so much better after that trip to the bathroom that my family even came up with a little dance for me. It was called the "Bathroom Victory Dance."

The *berachah* of *asher yatzar* took on a completely new meaning to me after experiencing chemo.

I told that to Dr. Harris and he gave me an article written by his friend, Dr. Kenneth Prager, M.D., who was a doctor at Columbia Presbyterian Hospital in New York. It was such an amazing and inspiring article that I stuck it into my journal so that I could always read it again.

Faigy, Yitzy, and I were all sick in bed over Shabbos, but by Motza'ei Shabbos I felt much better, so Miss Riegler came over to help me catch up on the math I was missing. We had a good time, even though I couldn't figure out how to use my graphic calculator for all the money in the world, and just ended up pressing random buttons for fun.

I was up until six in the morning because I was in a lot of pain and because my nose was bleeding constantly. My platelets were low and every time I sneezed, blood would come gushing out of my nose. It was also the time in my cycle where my hair would fall out and this time around my eyelashes and eyebrows were going. I was not very happy at all.

My night sweats and rashes were back and running between Yitzy and me, my mother didn't get much sleep that night either.

Sunday,
January 04 2004

For Everything a Blessing

by Kenneth M. Prager, M.D.
Columbia Presbyterian Medical Center, New York

When I was an elementary school student in yeshivah — a Jewish parochial school with both religious and secular studies — my classmates and I used to find amusing a sign that was posted just outside the bathroom. It was an ancient Jewish blessing, commonly referred to as the *asher yatzar* benediction, that was supposed to be recited after one relieved oneself. For grade-school children, there could be nothing more strange or ridiculous than to link to acts of micturition and defecation with holy words that

Reprinted with permission from Kenneth M. Prager, M.D.

mentioned G-d's name. Blessings were reserved for prayers, for holy days, or for thanking G-d for food or for some act of deliverance, but surely not for a bodily function that evoked smirks and giggles.

It took me several decades to realize the wisdom that lay behind this blessing that was composed by Abayei, a fourth-century Babylonian rabbi.

Abayei's blessing is contained in the Talmud, an encyclopedic work of Jewish law and lore that was written over the first five centuries of the Common Era. The Jewish religion is chock-full of these blessings, or *berachot*, as they are called in Hebrew. In fact, an entire tractate of Talmud, 128 pages in length, is devoted to *berachot*.

On page 120 (*Berachot* 60b) of the ancient text it is written:

> Abayei said, when one comes out of a privy he should say: Blessed is He who has formed man in wisdom and created in him many orifices and many cavities. It is obvious and known before Your throne of glory that if one of them were to be ruptured or one of them blocked, it would be impossible for a man to survive and stand before You. Blessed are You that heals all flesh and does wonders.

An observant Jew is supposed to recite this blessing in Hebrew after each visit to the bathroom. We young yeshivah students were reminded of our obligation to recite this prayer by the signs that contained its text that were posted just outside the restroom doors.

It is one thing, however, to post these signs and it is quite another to realistically expect preadolescents to have the maturity to realize the wisdom of and need for reciting a 1600-year-old blessing related to bodily functions.

It was not until my second year of medical school that I first began to understand the appropriateness of this short prayer. Pathophysiology brought home to me the terrible consequences of even minor aberrations in the structure and function of the human body, At the very least, I began to no longer take for granted the normalcy of my trips to the bathroom. Instead, I started to realize how many things had to operate just right for these minor interruptions of my daily routine to run smoothly.

I thought of Abayei and his blessing. I recalled my days at yeshivah and remembered how silly that sign outside the bathroom had seemed. But after seeing patients whose lives revolved around their dialysis machines, and others with colostomies and urinary catheters, I realized how wise the rabbi had been.

And then it happened: I began to recite Abayei's *berachah*. At first I had to go back to my siddur, the Jewish prayer book, to get the text right. With repetition — and there were many opportunities for a novice to get to know this blessing well — I could recite it fluently and with sincerity and understanding.

Over the years, reciting the *asher yatzar* has become for me an opportunity to offer thanks not just for the proper functioning of my excretory organs, but for my overall good health. The text, after all, refers to catastrophic consequences of the rupture or obstruction of any bodily structure, not only those of the urinary or gastrointestinal tract. Could Abayei, for example, have foreseen that "blockage" of the "cavity," or lumen, of the coronary artery would lead to the commonest cause of death in industrialized countries some 16 centuries later?

I have often wondered if other people also yearn for some way to express gratitude for their good health. Physicians especially, who are exposed daily to the ravages that illness can wreak, must sometimes feel the need to express thanks for being well and thus well-being. Perhaps a generic, nondenominational *asher yatzar* could be composed for those who want to verbalize their gratitude for being blessed with good health.

There was one unforgettable patient whose story reinforced the truth and beauty of the *asher yatzar* for me forever. Josh was a 20-year-old student who sustained an unstable fracture of his third and fourth cervical vertebrae in a motor vehicle crash. He nearly died from his injury and required emergency intubation and ventilatory support. He was initially totally quadriplegic but for weak flexion of his right biceps.

A long and difficult period of stabilization and rehabilitation followed. There were promising signs of neurological recovery over the first few months that came suddenly and unexpectedly: movement of a finger here, flexion of a toe there, return of sensation here, adduction of a muscle group there. With incredible courage, hard work, and an excellent physical therapist, Josh improved day by day. In time, and after what seemed like a miracle, he was able to walk slowly with a leg brace and a cane.

But Josh continued to require intermittent catheterization. I know only too well the problems and perils this young man would face for the rest of his life because of a neurogenic bladder. The urologists were very pessimistic about his chances for not requiring catheterization. They had not seen this occur after a spinal cord injury of this severity.

Then the impossible happened. I was there the day Josh no longer required a urinary catheter. I thought of Abayei's *asher yatzar* prayer. Pointing out that I could not imagine a more meaningful scenario for its recitation, I suggested to Josh, who was also a yeshivah graduate, that he say the prayer. He agreed. As he recited the ancient *berachah*, tears welled in my eyes.

Josh is my son.

Thursday, January 08, 2004

Regarding Blood and Burgers

Monday's chemo was okay, but as soon as I got home I developed a fever and was taken in to the emergency room.

Pinny threw a fit when my parents rushed out with me. He hated that I was getting all the attention. Pinny himself was quite the character and wasn't used to being sideswiped when it came to getting noticed. My father's friend, Shia Deutsch, had to come over and keep Pinny under control until we came home.

I was in the emergency room for about four hours until all

my bloods came back negative and my fever went down. After I had already picked out what room I wanted to stay in, the nurses came to tell me that I was going home.

I was so excited.

It was pretty late when we got home, and we thought we were going to come back to a sleeping house. We were kind of surprised when we walked in to find Faigy crying on the living room couch.

She was angry and hurt because a classmate of mine had called and asked her if she could talk to me. Faigy didn't want to say that I was in the hospital, so she told the classmate I was unavailable.

The classmate kept pushing Faigy around, trying to get her to hand the phone over to me and Faigy finally told her that I had been rushed into the hospital and that no one was going to get through to me that night.

Faigy said that my classmate wanted to know exact details and Faigy didn't think it was appropriate to tell her and besides, Faigy herself didn't know much, because by the time she came home from school that day we were already gone. She only knew what my parents told her when they called her every so often from the emergency room to check up on how things were going at home.

The girl asked Faigy if I was going to be okay and Faigy said she didn't have time to answer all her questions because she had a house full of kids that needed suppers, baths, and beds.

The girl then said to Faigy, "Wow, sounds like you really don't care about your sister."

Faigy told us that she got really upset then and started crying on the phone and told my classmate, "I don't care?! How dare you! I'm the one looking after all my siblings while my sister is sick, and I'm still trying to keep up with my schoolwork. *You're* the one who doesn't care enough to know when it's inappropriate to call and ask questions of people who don't owe you any answers!"

I thought my sister did a very good job in the way she handled that phone call and resolved to let her handle more of them for me. My father calmed her down and said she did the right thing, and that we were all sorry that things were getting so hard for everyone, and that people tended to pry into other people's business while still thinking it fell under the category of *chesed*.

Faigy felt a little better but was worried about how the girl would act toward her in school the next day. My mother said that she shouldn't think about it and that it didn't seem like the girl caught a hint fast enough to care about what other people thought and said about her. She probably didn't even realize that Faigy had shouted at her or that she had called at an inconvenient time.

After taking care of Faigy, we all, finally, went to bed.

I had to go back to the hospital the next day; Dr. Harris wanted me to be monitored because up until now, the ninth day of my chemo cycle was usually the day where everything went wrong.

He was right. I did get sick during the day, but the only thing they were able to do was give me laxatives and Benadryl. When I told them that I was taking the same things at home anyway, they let me go.

I finally started eating a little because while I was in the emergency room I had seen an ad there that showed a big, beautiful, juicy burger dripping fat and it made me so in the mood for one. I pestered my mother all day until I got one too.

It didn't taste as good as it had looked on in the ad, so I didn't finish more than a few bites.

My mother was already warning people that whoever married me was going to have a miserable time dealing with my cravings when I was going to be expecting one day.

Dr. Harris pointed out to her that by the way I had handled my last round of chemo, he was sure that anything else in life was going to be a breeze for me. I told him he was wrong. Pain was pain. Who cared which pain was stronger or easier or harder? When people are in pain, they don't want to hear how much harder or easier other people have it, they want their own pain to be acknowledged. He said I would make a good psychologist one day.

My cravings were caused by a steroid I was taking, called Prednisone. In three days I went from 92.8 lbs to 97 lbs. It could have been from all the fluids I was taking in with my hydration, but it made the doctors happy, so I didn't care where it came from.

I needed to go into Hackensack again on Wednesday because my lips were white and my moods were down. That probably meant my hemoglobin levels were low, which meant a blood transfusion was in order.

Yippee.

The hospital was storing blood my Uncle Dovid had donated for me, but I needed another pint in addition to the pint he gave. Even though we had tried to get all the blood I needed donated by people I knew, I had no choice here but to take a bag from an anonymous donor for this cycle.

The anonymous bag of blood came from the hospital blood bank and we were a little upset about it. We felt more comfortable getting blood from within the Jewish community, but the Monsey Bikur Cholim didn't have enough for me at that time.

Now I have a new blood relative that I need to find.

The nurses in the hospital were joking that it would make a great play: "The Search for My Biological Blood Donor."

My mother got on the task of getting my bloods lined up for my next cycle so that I wouldn't have to get any more anonymous blood. She felt that two anonymous blood relatives would kill the ratings of my potential hit show.

When Miri heard that we were looking for blood, she first wanted to know if I was going to bite her on the neck like a vampire. Then she wanted donate for me so that we could really be like sisters, but by that time I already had my bloods lined up for the next cycle and that was going to be my last, so I had to turn down her offer. In the end, my father's friend, Shia Deutsch, gave some and my last pint was from someone unknown as well, but taken from the Monsey Bikur Cholim bank.

Yossi and his father were going to donate just like Miri was, but I heard Yossi was very relieved when he found out that I had enough for my last round. My father told me that Yossi fainted every time he got a paper cut. I laughed for three days.

My stomach hurt that night but I had so much energy because of my new blood, so I called all my friends and stayed up late talking for hours. Except for the hydration, I felt almost normal.

Etty Gruen, the girl who warned me about chemo foods, cut school to come and visit me Thursday. She came to show me pictures and tell me about when she was sick. Dr. Harris was her doctor too, and we exchanged stories about what a mentch he was.

She bought me a pair of fuzzy slippers and a matching bandanna. I had given up wearing a hat in favor of bandannas. They were so much more comfortable, but now I really looked like I had cancer.

I was in isolation, my fingers were numb, my platelets were low, but I felt great. I had only one more round of chemo to go!

Abandonɛd

I was left to fend for myself Friday morning as most of the family packed up and left to the Chai Lifeline retreat in the mountains for the weekend. I wasn't allowed to join the fun and games and the swimming pool and the whole "meeting new people" experience because I was in isolation. Again.

Chemo was such a bummer.

As soon as I was alone with Yitzy and Nechama, we worked together to make a mess. Yitzy chased me around the house with a bottle of Windex, calling me "Hey, you!" while Nechama colored the walls with Crayola markers, humming happily.

About two hours before Shabbos, things began going crazy. I had to bathe and pack up the two little ones to go to my neighbor for Shabbos, and then I had to give myself my Neupogen shot. I was getting up my nerve to stick myself, when our pharmacist friend came over to help me out. That was a relief!

As I was settling into my next-door neighbor Leah Freund's house for Shabbos, Nechy Berger's parents called to tell me that they were kidnaping me for Shabbos. I appreciated their gesture so much, but I wanted to stay on the block near Yitzy and Nechama, because I knew how homesick they could get.

Finally, it was Shabbos. I ate and slept at the Freund's and it was really nice because it didn't feel like I was really away from home. I practically grew up in Leah's house, so it was just a regular Shabbos for me.

The whole time all Leah's sisters kept telling me how natural my sheitel looked and that if they didn't know I was sick they would never have guessed I was wearing one. It was flattering until one of Leah's nieces waltzed into the kitchen and asked me why I was wearing a sheitel.

If I hadn't burst out laughing, it would have been an embarrassing moment. I never bothered to pretend I didn't look sick. I knew I did. It was fine. Cancer is not an easy thing to hide. I did it the best I could and other than that I just had to accept that there were some things that were not in my hands.

Later that night, two of Leah's nephews began throwing up and it seemed that a stomach virus was going around. I tried to be good about my isolation thing, but I was only sixteen. I couldn't be expected to get it right all the time. I just hoped that I wouldn't get sick too.

After Shabbos I went home to find myself alone for the rest of the night. I didn't like that idea much so I called my friend Rikki Weber to pass the time. We passed the time until 5:30

in the morning. Then we went to bed until someone called my house and woke us up at eight. I think eight is way too early to call anyone on a Sunday morning.

For years my mother had been cooking suppers as a volunteer for Chai Lifeline. Every Sunday at four in the afternoon, like clockwork, a driver would pick up six suppers. If my mother knew that she wouldn't be home to prepare the suppers, she made sure someone was there to take care of them. So I spent that Sunday making supper for Chai Lifeline. I found that so ironic.

Once, our Chai Lifeline pickup guy saw me walking around the house in my bandanna and he asked my mother if we needed Chai Lifeline to send us suppers. My mother sort of looked at him while handing over the six meals she had just prepared and told him if she needed anything she would let him know, or she would just make the packages for herself.

My mother had done this for years already and didn't feel that she had to give it up just because I was sick. She felt that even though we were now on the receiving end of Chai Lifeline, there was no reason we had to stop giving.

When my family came home, my mother told me that at the retreat everyone was busy with the poem I had written, "He's Holding my Hand." I thought that was very nice. I liked the feeling that I was able to do something that inspired others.

My mother was repeating some of the things she had heard at the workshops during the retreat, and from what she said, it sounded like I missed out on a lot.

She mentioned that she had been sitting next to a very *choshuv* woman during a session about keeping your sanity while dealing with hardship, and that this rebbetzin had contributed what she did to stay normal. My mother imagined that this woman probably found solace and comfort in saying the whole *Sefer Tehillim* each day, but she was in for a shock and for a good laugh when the rebbetzin said that she had gone for a manicure.

My mother was ready to schedule a manicure for herself right then. The woman at the retreat said that there was only so much *Tehillim* you could say without going crazy, and that she also needed some *gashmiyus* time just for herself. She needed time to breathe.

I found it a cute story, but very real. Our minds were so wrapped around my Hodgkin's that it was hard to break away and do something else for a little while, even though we all needed it.

Later that night, to give me a break from my family, Suri Rubin came over and surprised me with a beautiful makeup set. She claimed I looked too pale and that I should spend my long days experimenting with makeup to try to make myself look healthier. She's the cutest!

Ayala called later that night and we schmoozed until midnight. My mother wasn't thrilled and threatened to make me stay home instead of going to school the next day, so I had to hang up in the middle of a very good conversation.

Ayala was just telling me that she had heard a *shiur* about people each having seven *zivugim* in life. Depending on what stage a person is in at a particular time, they have a *zivug* to match.

It was an interesting concept and it sort of made sense. I knew a few couples who had met and then decided they weren't for each other, only to get married five years later. It just meant that it wasn't the right time or stage for them the first go around.

I knew I was young, but I wondered what type of person I would end up marrying one day. As all-knowing sixteen-year- olds, Ayala and I both agreed that it was better to meet a *zivug* after you had been through some rough stages in life because then it would lead to a deeper relationship.

I love how we thought we knew everything about deep, meaningful relationships with our future husbands at sixteen. We all thought we were so intelligent. Well, we were, but that's another story ....

Wednesday,
January 14, 2004

The Teachers Who Shouldn't Be Teaching

*M*onday morning, I got into my uniform but as I was getting dressed, I discovered some huge bruises all over me, so that was the end of my school day. I had to rush to Hackensack for a blood count. Right off the bat they thought I would need a transfusion, but the bloods came back just above the platelet transfusion mark, so I was sent home.

On the way home (after we filled up on gas: $1.63), we stopped off to buy me some more bandannas. Then I got home and went to lie down, but I was too restless to fall asleep, and suddenly I found myself crying. It didn't help matters that the school play was going strong and I was missing out on all of it.

After my good cry, Faigy had one too. She had midterms coming up and she needed to make up some notes for classes she had missed, but none of her friends were home to help her because they were all in school for play practice. So I went to school in my bandanna and got some of her friends to give me their notes.

My mother went out with Chavy later because apparently, Chavy also had her own good cry that night. She was not happy about me taking over her whole *shanah rishonah*. Instead of her and Eli coming over for suppers, she was making the suppers for our family and she barely had time to experience married life.

I felt so bad to be the cause of everyone's good cry that night, but there wasn't anything I could do to be less of a burden on anyone. I was trying so hard to be good about it, but it made me feel so guilty anyway.

Pessie Miller came over to cheer me up later with a bunch of colorful bandannas and an adorable card that had everyone in stitches all night.

Tuesday, I finally made it to school. I skipped out on every boring period to join my friends in the sewing room where they were putting together costumes for the play.

Faigy came up to me to tell me she wasn't feeling well, and that she needed my help in getting out of school. She had never missed a day of school in her life and she didn't even know who the attendance administrator was. I was the old pro at this and took care of the whole thing.

I think that for all her complaining, she did miss having me around school.

Right around Minchah time there was an announcement over the loudspeaker that we should all say *Tehillim* for "So-and-So bas Plonis" because she had "*yene machlah*" and had been rushed into the hospital.

As everyone was taking out their siddurim all that came to my mind was, "Hey that happened to me last week!" I felt weird seeing how intensely the girls said *Tehillim* for that person. I appreciated that they said *Tehillim* for me too, but I didn't think of myself as that sick, and it was strange to see how others viewed my Hodgkin's.

It was almost the end of the day when a teacher passed me in the hallway and told me to take off my cap. She said, "Oh you girls in the play, you think you're so cool that you can run around in costumes all day. You'd better have a good reason for wearing a cap in my class."

I wasn't sure why she was so upset and told her my hat was to cover my sheitel.

She gave me a sarcastic smile and said I was adorable and didn't know my place.

Later, she walked into my class and when she saw me with the cap again, she got really angry. She started yelling about how the girls in the play thought they could mess up the whole school by wearing what they wanted and doing whatever they pleased.

She looked at my Delaney card in her folder for my name, and got even more upset when she saw that I had missed her classes for the last four months.

She went on to tell me, "And you think you can get away with cutting my class for four whole months and I'm not going to say anything about it? You've got to be kidding me; get out of my class."

I got up and told her, "I'm really sorry that it gets on your nerves that I have cancer and that I had to miss a bunch of your classes and need a wear a sheitel to school. If it bothers you so much, I won't come anymore."

My mother had just arrived to pick me up from school, so it was the perfect time for me to bow and make my exit.

Miss Riegler told me later that this teacher came into the office crying after I left. She felt so guilty about yelling at me and not knowing that I was ill.

Maybe I should have felt bad about making her cry, but I do believe it was her own fault. If she would have made the effort to get to know her students and find out what was wrong with a girl who had missed four months worth of classes, she could have neatly avoided that embarrassing spectacle and the expensive gift she bought me to make up for it.

School really knocked me out that day, so I left explicit instructions not to wake me until lunch the next day. Well, I was woken up for lunch, but it was for a nice surprise. My great-aunt Kayla Rubinstein came with her daughter Chaya to keep me company and make sure I ate something. I had a really nice time.

After they left, I spent the afternoon taking the Windex bottle away from Yitzy. My little brother kept trying to drink the Windex out of the spray nozzle, so I gave him blue Powerade in his bottle.

He was in Windex heaven.

Motza'ei Shabbos, January 17, 2004

Before my Next Round of Chemo

Thursday was a snow day and I couldn't believe it, but I actually had a great time with Faigy home to fool around with. She helped me make an explosion in the kitchen when we made challah for Shabbos together.

It was so much fun making the mess with an accomplice. I finally had someone to blame it on!

Friday morning my mother had an emergency at work, so she needed to go in even though the office was technically closed. Yossi Spitzer said he would drive me to my scans because he didn't have to go into work that day.

I was not especially happy, but I had no choice. I asked him to please wait in the car while I took care of my appointments. I didn't want him to come along and see all my scans.

Because it was Martin Luther King Day, I was wearing an American flag bandanna and a navy sweatshirt with a red stripe across it, and was off to Hackensack for a Pulmonary Function Test. It is the most uncomfortable, draining, stupid test that is a pain to take at any time of day, but is torture at a quarter to eight on a morning when the weather outside is three degrees Fahrenheit.

After the stupid test, I needed an echocardiogram. It was freezing sitting on the examining table in a hospital gown and then getting cold goo all over me. Ugh, it was so uncomfortable.

By ten, I was back at my parents' office building, where my father called me Baldy, and where everyone laughed at my patriotic bandanna until I ignored them all and went to take a nap in a corner somewhere.

That Sunday I was bored silly, so I convinced my mother to take me to a crafts store so that I could get started on our family Purim costumes. While I was there I got some paints and I was busy the rest of the night making Shmully a Bob the Builder yarmulke.

I spoke to Miri a little and listened to her hysterical story of how she left an open jar of herring in a locker at her school for a week and locked the door for fun, just to see what would happen. She said that they almost canceled school for the eleventh grade because the halls smelled so bad and they didn't know what was wrong.

It would have worked perfectly if Miri's name hadn't been on the padlock when they found out where the smell was coming from, and now she was suspended for a week, so if I wanted her company during chemo she was free to come along.

I laughed so hard, my port hurt. I didn't know whether to believe her or not, but when I called Michal to find out, I wasn't surprised to hear that most of it was true.

Miri and I did lots of pranks together, but she got along just fine in her school when I wasn't there.

Miss Riegler came over for a few minutes later to give me a $100 gift certificate to the music store and a HUGE poster board with a cute poem to celebrate my last round of chemo.

She's the best.

Miss Riegler's Poem

Hey you!
So I sat down and took the time,
To write you this heartwarming-kinda-rhyme.
Like, soon, soon, we're almost there,
And just from happiness I'm shedding tears!
The plan was all worked out and ready,
My pen was in my hand all sure and steady.
When the thought hit me like a rock,
And sent me reeling from the shock.
It was then that I was reminded,
Oh how was I so very blinded?
It was then that my brain went numb,

And I felt horribly incapable and dumb.
I'm sorry for this rhyming repetition,
It's just that I got totally afraid of the competition!
It was then that I remembered that ... YOU write,
And so I started feeling ever so small-n-slight.
So I let out a deep, deep sigh,
But imagined it couldn't hurt to try.
So sit back, spread your feet and toes,
This is MY poem; here goes!
One more round,
I like the sound
Soon you'll be over and done, the end,
Then all will be rosy, okay, student, friend?
'Cause it's just one more round,
And I like the sound.
You'll be strong and healthy and fit as a fiddle,
And there will be simcha in everyone, big and little.
'Cause it's just one more round,
Oh, how I like that sound!
Louis and David will vanish and die,
The happiness is so great; I must wipe my eyes.
'Cause it's just one more round,
What a wonderful sound!
So I figured, "What kind of gift, what matana,
Would adequately express, my happiness,
    my kavana?"
I figured I could buy you a good sefer; y'know
    the type,
Like "Hashem loves you," and "Pain makes you strong
    and ripe."
Then I imagined that you had your share of those,
So I continued pacing the aisles and rows.
Then I thought maybe a huge plush bear,

That takes up your chair and sheds white hair?
But I quickly abolished that notion,
And started thinking of makeup and lotion.
But I figured I might give you some time,
Before I cause you to commit some makeup crime!
   (After all I AM your teacher!!)
Then I went to the section with food,
And you can imagine what that did to my mood!
Every other item was "NAUSEOUS! DON'T EAT!"
I tell you, my mood was everything but upbeat.
I almost despaired,
When it miraculously appeared.
I thought I'd let you know it was the very last round,
By helping you fill your house and heart with sound!
Love,
Mindy Riegler

Monday, January 19, 2004

Last Round of Chemo!

Monday morning we started counting down my chemo medications. No more Cytoxin or Bleomycin anymore!

I told Dr. Harris that I might need to be on an antidepressant for a while because I was going to miss the clinic so much. Now he decided I should be a comedian. The man needed to make up his mind about what field he wanted me to go into.

People cannot understand what it felt like to finally be leaving the clinic. It really did feel depressing. The nurses and doctors had become our support group, our friends, and our family.

During chemo we were counting down until we got out of there, but when the time finally came, it was so hard to leave all the people who had come to mean so much to us.

We were anxious to get back to real life, but for the last year, the clinic *was* our real life. No one taught us how to go from one to another. It was a very hard transition, and on the way back to my old life, there was no support system like the one we had going in.

Even though it was the last time and we all felt great about it, chemo was still chemo and it made me feel awful.

Despite the way I felt, I convinced my mother to take me to the mall on the way back from chemo. She was hesitant, but I reminded her that she owed me a rain check from another time where she had offered and I declined.

I wore the hydration bag (not that I had a choice anyway), and my mother made me promise to tell her as soon as I wasn't feeling well so that she could take me straight home.

I didn't end up getting anything because manufacturers don't make things for teens who weigh less than fifth-graders, but my mother found something to wear for my brother Zevy's bar mitzvah! It was at a great price that even my father couldn't say anything about, but I'm not allowed to tell anyone what we paid. We were so excited the whole way home.

Sunday,
January 25, 2004

Just Finish Up
Already!

I started having night sweats again, and my IV kept beeping and I kept going to the bathroom all night, so I was not in a good mood on Friday until they de-accessed my port. After that I was finally able to take a decent shower and scrub my head, arms, and legs, even balder.

Somehow, in the rush before Shabbos, I forgot to take my GCSF shot. I was so excited. The shots hurt more and more with every cycle. By the time my fourth round came up, I was in so much pain, it hurt to even breathe. I didn't have to move in order to feel the pain; it was a constant ache in my very bones.

It's a hard pain to describe. It's a pain that comes from within a part of you that you didn't know you had. It hurts way inside the bones; a feeling that is very strange. It's like hearing the walls of a house creak; like the very structure of your body is complaining.

But when my father asked the *dayan* in shul what we should do, he insisted that I get my shot. He said there was no question about medical issues on Shabbos.

Bummer.

Because I had worn the hydration all week, I still had a lot of fluid in me and had to go to the bathroom very often, but I didn't mind it so much, because I wasn't going to have to wear the thing again until Monday. I knew I was getting a little dehydrated, but I didn't say anything for fear of being hooked up again to that infernal beeping pest.

But then my dreams of a hydration-free weekend were shattered when the home healthcare company informed me that they were going to come over right after Shabbos to hook me up.

My parents wanted me to be hydrated even before chemo on Monday. They were hoping it would keep me out of the hospital this round. I was so appreciative of how much they adored and cared for me, but this came at the expense of a good night's sleep and my personal dignity. I wasn't happy.

Shabbos afternoon Meira and Pessie came over to visit. As we were on the couch, we began tossing a ball around. I kept dropping it every time it came to me. Dr. Harris had warned me about losing some of my reflexes. I felt like an unsteady toddler. Between dropping balls and navigating stairs, I looked pretty stupid around people who didn't know what was wrong with me.

As we were schmoozing, the home health care company nurse rang the doorbell. She had come to access my port, fours hours early. I was far from thrilled.

My friends got to watch as the nurse stuck me and hooked me up to my beeping bag. They got to see part of what I did every day. I felt silly, but they were really interested in everything I had to do on a normal day of chemo.

Sunday, we stopped in the crafts store for a few minutes and those few minutes were an opportune time for my backpack to begin beeping. Loudly.

The store emptied quickly. I think people assumed I was wired to an explosive. Someone even yelled for security.

How to explain to a seven-foot security guard that I was a sixteen-year-old girl with cancer who had to wear a bag strapped to her back?

We got out of there before we could get into a really embarrassing situation.

I couldn't wait to be over and done with it all! One more day of chemo left!

Monday, January 26, 2004

Last Day of Chemo!

I was busy all Monday saying my goodbye's to every-one in the clinic. Sue, the child-life specialist, brought me a T-shirt printed with the clinic's logo, and we got everyone there to sign it. We stayed for a while even after my chemo was done so that I could snap pictures with every doctor, nurse, patient, chair, table, and IV pole that wasn't already in my scrapbook.

I was upset because I lost the entire roll of film that I took during my first round of chemo. That film had the pictures of my *upsherin* and of my first hospital stay. I was trying to take lots of pictures to make up for them.

I told Rachel, my advanced-practice nurse, about my film and told her that I thought I needed to be readmitted to the hospital for a while so that I could redo all the photos.

Rachel said I was *meshugah*.

We filled up on gas for what we hoped was the last time in New Jersey, and marveled at how the price per gallon had gone up to $1.65, more than twenty cents above what it had cost at the start of my cycles.

As soon as we hit the George Washington Bridge on the way home, my mother commented that my eyes were getting glassy and that she could see the fever coming. She wasn't imagining things. As soon as I got home, I crawled into my father's bed and took my temperature every fifteen minutes until it hit 101. Then I called to my mother to pack my bags and take me back to Hackensack.

I was feeling worse this time around than I had ever felt during any other cycle. I kept blacking out over and over again. I told my mother to keep the camera handy to snap a picture as soon as I went under again. It's the only picture in my scrapbook where I'm not smiling.

Because we knew that it would be my last time in the emergency room, my mother took a ton of pictures with everyone there. I was half-dead in all the shots, but I insisted my mother take the photos. There were enough nurses to take care of me while she worked on my scrapbook.

I finally got up to the Rocklin Building, where Joanne was my nurse for the night. I was pumped up with morphine and I was dead to the world until four in the morning, when Joanne came to take my vital signs and stayed to chat with me as I asked her a million questions.

Tuesday,
January 27, 2004

Bring the Food and
Eat It Yourself!

I was still pretty dead when my mother came to visit me on Tuesday with a full tray of little cups filled with different flavors of ice cream. I didn't want to eat anything, but she was hoping that I would be tempted by at least one of the flavors on the tray. She ate it all herself in the end, and then obsessed about it the whole day because she was worried about fitting into that beautiful new dress for the bar mitzvah.

I reminded her that it was at such a good price anyway, she could totally have gone back and gotten the next size, too, and the bill would still not amount to much.

I don't think that's what she wanted to hear, but she ate a few more spoons after that.

A group of kids from the Hackensack high school came to the ward to do their good deed for the day. A cheerleader named Kelly brought me a football and a volleyball because she heard from the nurses that I liked being active. Later, the captain of the track team, Joanne, and her friend, who was the captain of the soccer team, kept me company. Then they all had to leave, and so did my mother, so I was free to black out again.

The blacking-out thing went on for most of the night. I fainted while I was on the phone with Miri, Ayala, Devoiry, and then Miss Riegler. I finally buzzed the nurse and told her that I fell when I went to the bathroom and I was dizzy even when I was lying down.

The doctor decided to take me off the morphine and said that I wasn't allowed to get up, not even to go to the bathroom, without a nurse.

Dr. Harris wasn't happy that I had to be admitted to the ward. In my third cycle the hydration had managed to keep me out of the hospital, but it didn't work now. My hemoglobin was really low, so I got a blood transfusion Tuesday morning. I took a picture holding the bag of blood. It felt warm and yucky in my hands, but it meant my lips were white for the last time.

I tried eating, but everything came up. It was wonderful. I never felt so thin in my whole life. I was just touching 90 lbs. I think it was the only time I ever actually wanted to *gain* weight.

Thursday, January 29, 2004

Mazal Tov and Goodbye, Rocklin Ward!

Wednesday was a snow day even though it had only snowed about half-an-inch the night before. It had been a very mild winter that year, and the schools hadn't given that many snow days. I guess they felt bad about all that missed vacation so they shoved a snow day in to be nice.

Faigy came to see me in the ward for the first time since

I started chemo. She freaked out a little to see me in a large hospital bed, hooked up to so many machines. I tried getting her to sit near me on the bed so that we could take a picture, but she was afraid to come too close. It felt awkward.

Miss Riegler also came along for the day. I was still very dizzy and couldn't even sit up for too long, so I had to lie in bed most of the time she was there. She was also as spooked as Faigy was to see me with a bunch of machines.

Miss Riegler walked around the ward and became attached to a little boy named Abie who had been in the hospital practically since he was born because he had a brain tumor. Everyone who came up to the Rocklin Ward was taken with Abie. My grandfather loved him to pieces, too. He used to bring him toys every time he came.

When Miss Riegler wasn't in Abie's room, she was on her cell phone. She had some very important matters to attend to. She called me later that night to tell me she was engaged!

I was so happy for her! All my friends were happy too, but they didn't know why her getting engaged was so special compared to everyone else. Her *chasan* was a cancer survivor and didn't care at all that she was diabetic. He claimed that she was a big girl who knew how to take care of her condition and that diabetes that was under control was no reason not to marry a wonderful girl like her.

Of course my father still thought that Yossi was perfect for her, but by now even Yossi rolled his eyes when my father brought it up.

I had to hang up on all the *mazal tov* calls because I needed to vomit, but as soon as I threw down the phone, the hospital chaplain walked in and I had to hold it. I didn't think it was nice to puke in front of a rabbi.

He visited for a while and then as he was getting up to leave, I grabbed a bowl and threw up. He looked like he felt as bad as

I did, but I wiped my mouth and smiled as if I had just finished brushing my teeth.

He grinned back, but it was halfhearted.

The doctor on the ward walked in as the rabbi was leaving and told me that I was free to go home. I was so excited.

When my mother came, they told her that my white blood count was still low and that I needed to continue my Neupogen shots. We also learned that my platelets were still dropping, so I would probably need to take a blood count the next day to see if I needed a transfusion.

Splendid.

My mother was so thrilled when I said I wanted ice cream, so she went straight from the hospital to the nearest kosher restaurant to buy me some. After a spoonful I was nauseous, so I lay back on the backseat and slept the whole way home holding a cup of melted ice cream in my hands.

I felt lousy all night, partly because I was sick, and mostly because it was the night of the major dress rehearsal for the school play.

Motza'ei Shabbos, January 31, 2004

From Platelets to Play

Bright and early Friday morning we were on our way to Hackensack for a CBC. Ann the PA came in to tell us that my results were not great, but still above the transfusion level.

I insisted that I needed platelets because I had never done it yet and it was already my last round of chemo and I wasn't going to get another chance to add it to my scrapbook. She thought I was being funny.

While I was wrangling my terms with her, I sneezed and sprayed blood all over myself. Ann told me that was the reason I had to cover my mouth and nose when I sneezed. It was just in case a geyser of blood decided to shoot out.

I wasn't sure if she was convinced yet, so I showed her how I was able to gather enough blood in my throat after a sneeze to gargle it.

Ann ran to get me the platelets.

Of course we took lots of pictures, but it was really different than getting blood. The stuff in the bag was white and sticky-looking instead of dark red.

Guess what? We got to fill up on gas in New Jersey again!

Friday night I cried for a good few hours because I wasn't in the school play. Chavy and Eli were eating the meal at our house and Chavy was so bratty to me. She kept saying that now that chemo was over I was just upset about losing all the attention so I had to find something else to cry about.

She made me feel so sick; I went to bed at 7:30 and didn't wake up until eight the next morning.

After Shabbos Pinny decided to murder me and sat on my head until my parents came home to rescue me.

I am so blessed to have a brother like Pinny.

Fighting with Pinny had knocked me out, so I took an Ambien and tried to go to bed, but then the Landers asked me to babysit so I dragged myself there instead.

I got back way past midnight, but my mother was still up doing my cancer scrapbook. She had just finished the page on which she had put a picture of her sticking my arm with the Neupogen needle. At the top of the page she had written, "Give me a ..." and then made four little cheerleaders holding signs, each carrying one letter of GCSF.

We were laughing hysterically over that page until two in the morning.

Sunday, February 01, 2004

Is Life a Play?

It was nothing new that I felt horrible all Sunday. The Neupogen was killing me. It was coming from deep within my bones. It wasn't a pain I could put an ice pack on to soothe, it was a deep intense pain that came from depths I didn't even know I had. And it got worse with every cycle of chemo.

By the time I had reached the end of my fourth cycle, the shots were so painful that I was in tears almost all day. I had to take codeine liberally.

When Sunday came around, codeine wasn't helping anymore. I figured that if I was in pain and crying anyway, I might as well go on over to the school play and see what was going on.

I wore my Clyde sheitel, and so many people had to look twice to see if it was my hair or not.

Now that Miss Riegler was getting married, she was looking into sheitels too. We had a big discussion about whether or not the wigs that looked so natural were the "right" thing or not for a married person. We knew that for a cancer patient it was the best thing ever, but for a married woman, was it right to look as if she wasn't even covering her hair?

I was glad I had a while before I had to worry about things like that. For me, Clyde was the greatest thing since sliced bread, or peanut butter, or grilled cheese, or whatever it is that people out there like.

I wasn't as jealous as I had expected to be when I watched the play. I got bored in the middle and went up to fool around in the lighting room with Devoiry.

Towards the end of the play, Meira and I ended up alone at the end of a quiet hallway, and we sat and talked on the floor there. I tried telling her that I really wasn't that upset about not being in the play, but I still cried.

At that point I honestly didn't want to be in that play. It was just that being there made me sad. I think I realized then that my life was more dramatic than any play could ever be. I played the game every day. I smiled when I felt awful, pretended things were okay, and stayed strong when I felt like giving up.

I left the play that night knowing in my heart and mind that my life was the play in which I took center stage and that no one could take that from me. Cancer just made my act more interesting and challenged me to be the actress I claimed to be.

My night didn't get better when I had to drink a full bottle of that melted taffy stuff for my CT scan the next day. It goes without saying that we took a lot of pictures of all the funny faces I made. I turned the most beautiful shade of green that would put any witch to shame. I considered auditioning for the remake of the Wizard of Oz while I was still in play mode ....

Tuesday, February 03, 2004

Horrible Drinks Are Worth It for a Concert!

I thought I was going to die in the car on the way to Hackensack Monday morning because I was so crazy nauseous. Somehow I made it to the clinic where Debra the nurse threaded an IV through my hand and taped it down on a board for my CT scan. I drank another cup of the horrible stuff and then it was off for a chest x-ray where we, of course, took pictures.

I cried while we waited an hour-and-a-half for my CT scan. I hadn't been allowed to eat anything except for the taffy drink since the night before, and I wasn't able to eat anything until after the scan. I almost threw up the last eight ounces of the contrast drink, but my mother warned me that if I did, she was going to make me drink another whole bottle.

That thought almost made me puke again.

After the long-awaited scan, it was back to the clinic so that Dr. Thomas, the neurologist, could investigate the cause of the severe headaches I'd been experiencing. He said that they were most likely from the GCSF shots and suggested that I take Advil.

Advil! Gee, why didn't I think of that?

I had planned to go to school on Tuesday, but I felt so horrible that I just ended up staying home. Morah Templer came to visit and she brought over an ice-cream cake and champagne to celebrate my ending chemo. She had waited until the end of the round because she knew I wouldn't have been in the mood to eat earlier.

Later that evening, Rikki Weber and Malky Gold called to tell me that they had somehow gotten me free tickets and backstage passes to an upcoming concert by my favorite singers. I was too excited to even talk, so I danced around instead. I was jumping for a week-and-a-half.

Pinny was so jealous!

MWAHAHAHAHAHAH! (evil laugh)

Am I Invisible, or Are You Just Stupid?

*J*schlepped my cancer scrapbook to school on Wednesday, aiming to show it off. I covered all the pictures of my bald head with Post-It notes, but everyone asked to see them anyway.

I was having a great day up until my favorite class came up; Public Speaking. We sometimes had to give speeches as part of our grade, but mostly the class was all about discussion. We were marked based on our participation and how much we contributed to the discussion of the day.

The discussion was usually started by our teacher reading

an interesting article or poem out loud to the class, and then we all voiced our opinions on it and were allowed to go as off-topic as we wanted, as long as we kept the discussion going.

That day's discussion topic was hardship.

The class was very moved by the article our teacher read and then the teacher asked the girls what kinds of hardships came to mind.

I wasn't expecting anyone to say cancer or illness because I was sitting right there, and I expected a certain amount of common sense and shyness around me and my sheitel. I also didn't want my class talking about cancer when I was there because I was sure I'd feel very stupid if they did.

It was just fine. No one even thought to bring up anything like it. Instead, the hardships discussed that day were even more stressful than I could ever imagine.

A girl raised her hand and told the teacher, "Well, right now we are all going through a really stressful time and we don't know how to handle it."

I was sitting a seat away from her and wondering what in that little brat's life could be so stressful, when she continued. "We're taking midterms next week and we are all so pressured!"

Life's biggest challenges were midterms. Yeah, right ....

The teacher started talking about perspective, about how a good attitude could turn even the hardest life experiences around, and blah blah blah, so I raised my hand to contribute. I told her about a girl in my hospital whose mother had taken her there to be diagnosed but was afraid of her playing in the playroom with all the bald kids. She was afraid her daughter would be traumatized.

At the end of the day, on the way home, she asked her daughter what she had thought of the kids there. Her daughter looked up at her and said, "Those kids are the luckiest kids in the world! They have the coolest toys in the playroom and get to have fun all day!" She hadn't even noticed the bald heads.

The mother pointed them out to her and the girl just shrugged and said, "Even cooler, they never have to take a shower because no one ever knows when their hair is oily!"

I was so turned off by that class.

Here I was, bald, sick, trying to cope, and there they were; talking about midterms being the hardest challenge for them to overcome. I was peeved, I was glad for them that they led such shallow lives and never had anything worse to cry about, but that stung, it really did.

A Week of Randomness

*P*inny met the producer of the upcoming concert in shul that Friday night and went right over to him to tell him that his sister had gotten free tickets to his upcoming concert and that he wanted some too.

The producer explained to Pinny that the only free tickets he knowingly gave out were to a sick girl and her friends. He told Pinny that I probably got the free ticket because my friend was sick and I wanted to take her out to make her feel better.

Pinny made a face at him and told him it wasn't true. He said I didn't have any friends that were sick. The producer was looking a little angry and confused, when Zevy told him quietly that I was the sick one and not my friend.

Mr. Producer wasn't able to say anything more than "Oh" after that.

He did tell Pinny that if my friends would call requesting a ticket for him too, then he would give him one. Pinny knew better than to think I was going to let him tag along on my night out with friends, and didn't bother asking me. He sulked all Shabbos.

It was a good thing he didn't ask, because if he did my parents would have asked me to take him, and I would have felt guilty enough to say *yes*.

It felt so nice to have finally won a battle with Pinny.

It felt nice until Motza'ei Shabbos when I went to see the school play again.

As soon as I walked into the auditorium, I bumped right into a teacher from my school. Before even telling me hello, she asked me to turn my baseball cap around to the front.

I only wore a cap to keep my sheitel from sliding off my shiny head, and I wore it backwards out of convenience. Wearing it the right way blocked my vision and it drove me crazy.

It was bad enough wearing a wig without the comments, but this was too much for me, and then to make it worse, my mother told me I had to listen to the teacher.

She claimed that while I was at the play I was setting an example and that it wasn't nice to give people an impression of their students that my school didn't want to project.

She was right, but I had enough, so I spent my time out of sight in the lighting room, and kept my cap firmly in place — backwards.

My night got worse when, on the way home, Faigy couldn't stop talking about how great the actress who got the main part in the play was. That was the part I had wanted. That was the part I worked for and almost got. I didn't need to hear how well other people were doing performing the part that was meant for me. It hurt enough that I wasn't in it. Did we all have to shove it in my face by praising the girl who had gotten the part I'd wanted ever since I was in pre-school?

In real life I never complained this much. That's why I had to keep this journal. Most of what I felt was put down here and no one ever had to know it.

Whatever.

In other news: Chai Lifeline had organized a trip to Disney-world sometime in January: it was the day after the retreat in the mountains that my family had gone to when they abandoned me for Shabbos. I missed both the retreat and Disney because I was in isolation.

Judy arranged a ski trip for some of the teens who were treated at Hackensack. After a lot of consideration, and a lot of trust in me, my parents agreed to let me go along.

I could barely sleep Tuesday night because I was so excited and nervous.

Ski Trip

arly Wednesday morning my mother drove me to Hackensack to meet the other eight kids going up to Hunter Mountain on the ski trip. They ranged in age thirteen to twenty-one, and I was the only one of them wearing a skirt. Everyone else on the trip had hair too; I was the only bald one with a bandanna. I was also the only Jewish kid there.

The ride up to the mountains was awkward. The rest of the kids all knew each other and I was kind of shy.

Sue Daniels came along on the trip and she kept me company until I warmed up to the others.

It took a few hours to get up to the lodge, where we met the couple who sponsored the trip and ate lunch with them.

I didn't eat too much even though special kosher food was packed just for me.

When the time came to go skiing, all the other kids were so excited, but I was scared. I had no idea how to ski and I was freezing cold. I was watching little kids zoom down the mountain and listening to the kids talk about going down Black Diamond slopes, and all I could think of was how scary the bunny slope looked.

Nancy the PA had brought along her little daughter's ski stuff for me and I was walking around in her ten-year-old's bright pink-and-purple gear all day. I got two ski instructors of my very own who were so great. Within-half-an hour I was off the bunny slope, without poles, and racing all the rest of my group down the intermediate runs.

It was just like rollerblading, only I had to invert my ankles, where in blading, it's just the opposite. In the beginning I kept falling down and zooming down the mountain on the seat of my ski suit, but then I got better and made it all the way down still on my feet.

I decided that the next time I was up there skiing, I would try snowboarding instead. It looked like a lot of fun until I watched some show-off land on his head. I tried to turn around to see if he was okay, but then I landed smack in a snowdrift ... again.

At three in the afternoon we got back into the bus and went to a snow-tubing place nearby. I didn't win any races down the hill because I wasn't heavy enough to get my tube even half-way down. Finally, I got three of the girls to join me in a pile and we managed to get it going.

After a while I learned how to make it work for me. I placed the tube at the top of the hill and then ran about ten feet back and cannonballed into the tube to send it zooming. I did it two or three times before I tried cannonballing and missed my tube and saw stars for a long time.

Nancy the PA and another nurse went down so fast that their tubes didn't stop at the bottom of the hill. Instead, the inertia of their tubes sent them flying up another small hill until they crashed into the gate that encircled the property and got stuck. It was so hilarious to us, but the nurses were really embarrassed.

After we were all tired out, we got back to the ski lodge to eat supper. We were allowed to order drinks as long as they were nonalcoholic, and one of the girls was very busy trying to get me to drink some drink with a weird name. I tried telling her that I wasn't sure if I could have it because I didn't know what was in it and I wasn't sure if it was kosher.

She wanted to know if kosher was some kind of allergy.

I soon had eight kids and a bunch of staff members around me while I tried to explain what kosher was.

They asked me a load of questions that I had no idea how to answer. I was sixteen, and they all expected me to have *semichah*!

During supper we were all overtired and hyper and I taught everyone how to hang spoons from their noses. The nurses took a lot of pictures of me smiling hugely behind a spoon dangling from my nose.

After all was eaten and cleared, we were taken to the prettiest bed-and-breakfast place. I couldn't get over how stunning it was. There were the sweetest little rooms that were all decorated differently, and the whole place had an old-country type of feel. The hosts were a sweet old couple who were so good to us.

As tired as we were, we were up all night bouncing around and playing games. The kids were all eating chocolate and I couldn't have any because I was *fleishigs*. They understood why I didn't want to mix milk and meat, but not why I had to wait six hours. That set off another round of explaining.

After the board games, the girls had a slumber party. They were all talking about their schoolfriends and things. When it came to my turn to join the conversation I told them what it was like to be in an all-girls' school and how life was fulfilling and fun.

The girls couldn't believe that I didn't have any friends that were boys, so to save face, I told them about David and Louie. Of course they all thought it was hilarious when they found out where David and Louie lived, and it was funny enough that they forgot to bombard me with some more rabbinical questions.

I left for a minute to go to the bathroom and as I came back saying *asher yaztar*, the girls wanted to know who I was talking to.

I blushed and said I was talking to G-d, thanking him for letting my body function properly.

One girl asked if it were okay to talk to G-d about bathroom stuff and those types of things. I asked her who she thought created that part of her, and she was like, "Oh."

Another girl asked why I had to thank G-d. I asked her if she ever had Vincristine as part of her chemo package. She nodded and said she remembered the pain it put her in.

I told her that I remembered it too and that every time I was able to go I thanked Hashem for making it a natural process and not something I had to cry for. I explained that I thanked Hashem for every second that I was healthy.

The girls wanted to know if they were allowed to pray that prayer too … and if my G-d would mind listening to them if they weren't Jewish.

Now how to answer that one?

As the party was coming to a close, I went into a corner and started to say *Shema*. Of course that sparked another discussion.

I was asked if it was okay to talk to G-d just like that. Did He hear me when I just talked even though I wasn't in a church? I told her that I would have called Him on my cell phone but there was no service. She made sure to ask me a million times if I was joking. I guess being Jewish was so foreign to her that she never knew when to take me seriously or not.

By seven the next morning we were up and eating breakfast at the lodge. I ate a banana and licorice and a chocolate bar and then was off to the slopes.

I was looking forward to doing a harder slope that day, but right away I saw I had a problem. As soon as I strapped on my skis, my left knee started buckling under me. My knee was always weak and because I had worked so hard on skis the day before, I couldn't stand very well, much less ski that morning.

I was put in a bi-ski where I was able to go skiing sitting down. It was terrifying. A bi-ski doesn't let you have as much control as regular skis give you. Someone had to ski behind me holding my chair on a leash so that they could help me stop. I kept tumbling out of the bi-ski and gave up after twenty minutes.

I waited around until after lunch when all of us got to take a lift to the top of the mountain. I was scared to death, but it was worth it. It was so amazing and beautiful. At the top we saw the Black Diamond slopes and I almost fainted with dizziness looking down at how steep they were. I would not try a Black Diamond even going down sitting.

When we chose to come down from the top, we all got to take wild rides on snowmobiles. *Cool* was not the word.

We said our goodbyes to the instructors and got a bunch of souvenirs and sweatshirts and hugs, and then got on the bus and slept most of the way home.

With about an hour left to our trip, we all woke up and started acting hyper. I was listening to a CD by my favorite Jewish band, and one girl asked to hear it. She was a black girl and she was bouncing away to the songs and trying to sing along to the Hebrew words. She wanted to know if she was allowed to walk into a Jewish store and buy the CD.

The other girls wanted to know what the songs meant. I explained that it was simple; all Jewish songs have one of three themes. They are either about marriage, family, or the praise and glory of G-d.

One of the girls wanted to know why there weren't any about love, like all her favorite songs, and another girl piped up to remind her that we Jewish gals didn't have boyfriends.

I must say I was proud of how quickly they had learned!

It was funny; a few weeks later that same singing group produced another album and every single song on the CD fit one of my three themes. It had me in stitches.

When I got home I talked all night, telling anyone who wanted to listen about my trip.

The black girl who liked my music was a liver cancer patient who kept relapsing no matter how many times she tried chemo. She had recently decided not to take any more chemo and just live her life as long and as happy as she possibly could.

The doctors had given her two weeks and she was okay with it.

I shouldn't judge her because I never went through anything like what she did, but I couldn't understand how someone could just give up. I thought everyone saw life as something precious. Why would she stop fighting if there was still a chance?

I was so happy I was not in her position and that I was on the way to remission. I never wanted to have to make the kind of choice about life that she did.

I was exhausted after jabbering on for hours and after dealing with my siblings who took apart all the souvenirs I got, and by the time I made it to bed, I was too tired to even get undressed.

Sunday, February 15, 2004

Concert!

had never gone to a real live concert with my friends before, and I was so hyped up all day about it. I got dressed about five times before I was happy with how I looked. Then I did my makeup for an hour-and-a-half. It took another fifteen minutes to arrange the cap on my sheitel just right, and then I waited for my friends to arrive.

I didn't believe it was all real until we gave our tickets in at the booth and were taken to our front-row seats.

Rikky Weber and Malky Gold and Etty Gruen were all with me. I had invited Faigy to come along, but she didn't care all that much for my favorite singing group. Pinny would have taken her place had I not locked him into the electrical closet earlier that day to keep him from following me.

Don't worry; no one missed him until he was discovered three days later by some Con Ed guy who came to read the meter. (Kidding ....)

My friends and I loved our amazing seats and we sang along to all the jumpy songs and waved our lighted cell phones to the slower ones, and did what all the other fans were doing: making complete fools of ourselves.

When the concert was over, my friends and I went backstage where we met the producer of the group. Right away he recognized me as the "sick girl" and told me that I had one monster of a brother.

He got all into it and called all the performers over so that I could meet them and get their autographs.

One of the guys asked me where I was treated and I told him Hackensack. He said he lived right there and that if we ever needed anything when I was inpatient, we should give him a call and he'd run over with whatever we needed.

I thought that he was such a mentch for offering. I was totally expecting all of the singers to be big-headed superstars, but they were all so normal and surprisingly nice.

I couldn't thank my friends enough for such a great night. It was a great way of celebrating the end to my four rounds of chemo.

As for Pinny .... It's been years and he still hasn't forgiven me.

Monday, February 16, 2004

WhεrΣ to Go From HΣrΣ?

I was all mixed up over the next few days. I was officially all better, and even though we didn't know yet if I would need radiation, I had to decide about going back to school.

Not that there was much of a choice. What else was a sixteen-year-old girl to do?

The problem was (and call me a snob if you will) that over the past four months I had changed so much that I dreaded going back to school and sitting in the same room with the grade mates who were still stuck on the everyday ins and out and politics of teenage life. I was so beyond that stage, I knew I would never be able to fit in again.

It wasn't like I was a little kid who could easily adjust to regular life again; I was a teenager who had been forced to become an adult in a very short time. I didn't feel like going back to being a teen now that I was well.

I didn't even think of blaming my grade mates for the way they acted. That was the way they were *supposed* to be acting. I was the different one. I had changed, not them. I had to decide whether I could handle sitting in class with girls who wouldn't like me once I didn't have Hodgkin's anymore; with girls whose hardest challenges in life were somewhere between Hebrew midterms and English ones, and whose high-school problems didn't really interest me.

I knew I couldn't.

My only question was; "So now what?"

I thought I might graduate early and get a head start in seminary or college, but I couldn't decide if that was what I really wanted. I was still slightly afraid that I would make the decision to leave school and then regret it when my friends were having a blast being seniors and goofing around. I couldn't decide if I wanted to grow up faster or try to be a kid again.

I had already taken some of my Regents exams on my own and I had no problem finishing the twelfth grade exams too so that I could graduate that spring. Miss Riegler was all for the idea, but I was afraid of giving up on fun I might lose out on. What fun? I didn't know. But I was still not sure if I was okay going in a brand-new direction.

Of course my father said that if I found a nice boy to marry, it would solve all my problems.

Parents! Sigh.

Tuesday, February 17, 2004

Finishing It All Up

*M*y PT scan would have been nothing to write about if the power hadn't gone out twenty minutes before I was done. The technician had to manually get me out of the machine and we had to wait until they reset the circuit breaker and then retake the last two parts of the scan.

I asked the tech what they did when a person who was three hundred pounds needed a PT scan. The hole in the machine didn't look that big. Funnily enough, he told me that anyone over three hundred-fifty pounds wasn't allowed to take the scan; otherwise they would get stuck in what I called the doughnut hole.

I assured him that I wasn't even a third of the way to three hundred lbs. He winked and said, "No kidding."

After the scan I visited the clinic to find out why I was having night sweats again. It turned out that my hormones were out of control; a regular short-term side effect of the chemo.

I had only finished chemo two weeks before, and already I was beginning to forget what life was like as a patient. I started feeling a little bit lost and left out of everything. I didn't feel like I belonged in the hospital anymore, but I didn't feel ready to go back to regular life.

It was back to that same debate. It was on my mind constantly over the next few weeks.

Motza'ei Shabbos, February 21, 2004

Remission!

*T*hursday, Dr. Harris called me on my cell phone to tell me that I had been randomized not to have to take radiation, so that meant that as of his phone call, I was in remission!

He said he wanted to give me the news himself because he said if he knew me at all, if a nurse had called I'd be ringing the office back demanding to hear the news from him anyway.

Even though I was now in remission, I still had to take a medication called Bactrim for a while. It was meant to protect my lungs from some aftereffects of chemo, but other than that, I was done. Finished.

The sound of that diagnosis was so beautiful to me. No radiation! We had been waiting to hear those two words since I started chemo.

When I came downstairs to the kitchen, I found my mother and father crying on the phone with Ann, my PA. Dr. Harris had called me personally with the news while his PA called my parents on the other line.

Did I mention what a mentch my doctor was?

During the whole time I was sick, my parents didn't cry like they cried that night. They were so relieved and happy after that phone call from Ann; all the emotions that they were too busy to deal with until now, finally came through.

We all hugged and laughed and cried together and my little siblings joined in. Of course, Yitzy might just have been crying because it was past his bedtime, but no one noticed.

No one can imagine what it was like inside my house that night. The younger kids didn't know what remission was, but they understood that it meant Mommy would be home more and that my hair was going to come back soon.

Chavy was happy to be a newly married wife again, while Faigy was excited to get back to being a regular teenager. Zevy was thrilled with the attention he was going to get for his upcoming bar mitzvah, and Pinny was jealous of Zevy now instead of me.

Dovid and the younger ones were just happy because we were happy.

My father went and called his friends to tell them that he had done a *shidduch* with someone named "Reb Mission." This is the kind of thing only a father of teenage daughters can do.

His friends were all happy for us, except for Yossi, who totally didn't get the joke. He asked my father how he could do a *shidduch* if his next in line was only sixteen. He was slightly confused until my father spelled it out for him.

Yossi apologized for being so slow, and wished us a huge *mazal tov*.

Shmully, my brother, told me that now that I was well I had to get buried. He meant married. I think he's been hanging around my father for too long.

I told him he had to find me a boy to marry and then I would gladly oblige. First, Shmully told me to marry my father. Then, when I explained to him that I needed a man who wasn't a Tatty yet, he told me to marry Zevy. When I explained to him that I couldn't marry my brother, he started setting me up with his classmates.

When I told him I needed to marry someone who was older than five, he told me he would have to think about it some more, but that he thought it would be a good idea if I stopped being so picky.

Oh, is he going to be some *shadchan* one day!

That Friday night when my father came home from shul, he and my brothers started dancing around the table while singing *Shalom Aleichem*. All of us joined hands and danced along. We came very close to crying again.

It was a pancake syrup kind of moment. You know, mushy and sweet and nice, but with no artificial sweeteners.

I went to shul on Shabbos and felt silly when I noticed all the ladies peeking over their *siddurim* to whisper about me. I had never gone to shul since I started wearing my wig, and I felt really self-conscious. I spaced out a little while the men were *leining* and then I snapped back in when I heard my name being read during a *mishebeirach* for a *refuah sheleimah*. Ohhh, that was embarrassing.

One lady, who had been obviously staring at me during the whole *Musaf*, came over to where Faigy and I were to ask which one of us was the sick one.

I was a little offended and wasn't very nice to her.

She felt bad right away and said that the only reason she asked was because she couldn't tell who was wearing the sheitel. I was slightly mollified, but still didn't know who she was.

She kept on talking about how she had heard so much about me and how she was so excited to meet me and that I was so much cuter in person and that I hardly looked sick at all.

I think after a while she realized that I had no idea who she was, and she introduced herself as Mrs. Spitzer. Oh. That felt so weird.

Faigy thought it was hilarious that Yossi had told his mother all about me and she giggled until Mrs. Spitzer said she had heard all about how Faigy was the paranoid one who was scared of failing her midterms.

Then it was my turn to laugh.

After shul we walked over to the Deutsch's house where I sat at the table and kept my mouth shut because I had nothing to say. My siblings went to play with the Deutsch kids, while the adults were talking at the table. I felt like I had to sit at the table because I was too old to run off and play, but I was bored because the adults were discussing their kids and it wasn't my kind of conversation.

My brother Shmully entertained everyone by telling them that I was looking to marry someone who was at least five years old if not older and that I was way too picky.

I didn't find it funny.

My day got even more annoying when my grandparents came over after Shabbos while I was wearing a bandanna. My father made me go upstairs and change into a sheitel, but I finally put my foot down. I wasn't going to put on an itchy sheitel in the middle of the night just because my grandparents came to drop in on my personal life.

I won this time. I had the bandanna on my head all night. Life was great.

Thursday, February 26, 2004

Reality Check

The excitement of remission had barely died down before midwinter vacation was over and it was back to school. This time I was going back with everyone else, as a regular student.

Okay, I wasn't really all that regular, I was wearing a sheitel and I was still weak and couldn't sit through an entire day of school and I missed out way too much work to really keep up in any class but Math, but for all anyone knew, I was a normal kid again.

My parents had worked it out with the school that I wasn't to be made responsible for any work until I felt ready to keep up with all the material. Right from the beginning I began working hard. I took it two subjects at a time and tried my best to catch up.

It was really weird for both Miss Riegler and me that I was her student again. We were friends. It was such a strange feeling to raise my hand in her class and to wait for her to call on me.

Some teachers decided they had their own opinions of how to make me fit in again. They bombed me with makeup work even though they had specifically been asked not to. Those teachers decided that I could do so much more than I was getting away with. One teacher even told me to write her a six-page report because I had missed her midterm.

Ugh. As if.

School made me so tired. I couldn't begin to think about homework when I got home. The only classes that I did well in at the beginning were Math, English, Chemistry, and Public Speaking, because those were classes that I was naturally good at.

Right after the midwinter break, we all had to give speeches in Public Speaking class. I gave one on how to administer a GCSF shot. I brought in four different types of needles and a GCSF bottle and a plum to stick. I had a great time sticking the needles into that fruit. It was so therapeutic.

The class didn't really know how to react. I think most people expected me to just forget and erase the last four months from my life. They didn't realize how much it had changed and affected me.

Michal said that she identified with the way I felt. She told me about a funny experience she had the year before, about the same time she had been starting radiation therapy. Some girls in her chemistry class insisted that people who took radiation glowed in the dark. They claimed that the radiation did something to patients' skin and that years later you could totally tell if a person had been through radiation once because they sort of glowed.

Michal had just begun taking radiation and was tempted to get up and shut the lights and see if she really glowed. She said that she felt so weird sometimes sharing her days with girls who really thought that way, and then wondered what she was gaining by keeping it all under wraps.

I agreed, but insisted that if she hadn't kept it secret, the girls probably would have shut the lights to see what parts of her lit up with the lights out.

That Shabbos my friend Suri Rubin took advantage of my fame by asking me to be a "guest speaker" at her class *shalosh seudos*. She was hosting the party and needed a speaker or else her school was going to send a teacher down to speak. She didn't need a teacher ruining her party, so she assured the school she had someone to talk; she just left out the part about me being sixteen.

Suri wanted me to talk about the petty stuff her class was into; like designer clothing and following the popular girls. She wanted me to talk to them about treating people like people and not like dirt just because they were different. Suri decided that with the sheitel on my head, I was qualified to give that speech.

I talked to the girls about my illness and said that I had no idea that one day the tables were going to turn on me. I had my whole life planned and suddenly, with my diagnosis, things changed drastically. It wasn't up to me where my life would end up, but what I did have control over was how I treated other people and how they could remember me.

It was funny, I was so beyond designer clothing and being popular, I almost forgot these things existed.

As soon as I got back into school, I was in for a reality check. Of course those things existed. My classmates didn't change just because I had. Now that I wasn't a celebrity any-more, it was back to whispering behind my back again by the girls in groups I didn't belong to.

I tried not to let myself care too much about it. I didn't want to waste my time caring about things I couldn't change. I went through things I hoped they'd never know, and I came out of them a stronger and better person. If they wanted to stick to their own lives and never try to see further into what they could do and become, it wasn't my business.

I had other important things to deal with. I got calls from just about every frum school in the tri-state area wanting me to talk to some student or other who had just been diagnosed with some form of cancer.

I always felt guilty when I got those calls. I had it so easy compared to others. My cancer had a 98% survival rate. Even though, as Michal said, the chemo was just as bad, I never had to live with the knowledge of potentially not making it.

I never said no when it came to giving *chizuk* to others, but I felt a little stupid doing it.

Once, when I was in a feeling-stupid kind of mood, my mother came home to tell me that a client of hers just lost her daughter to Hodgkin's. Michal was over at my house then, and when she saw I was so shocked, she asked me what was wrong.

"I thought there's a 98% survival rate!" I protested.

"Yes," Michal assured me, "but she was one of the two per-cent."

"But, I thought ...."

"It's like I told you when we met," she continued, "the sur-vival rates aren't everything. What we go through together is."

I was sad for my mother's client, and I never felt relaxed about my 98% survival rate again. Cancer was terrible, no matter which way you put it; no matter how assured you thought you were going to survive, only Hashem knew how it was going to end up.

Anyway, as busy as I was with the new life I had been shoved into because of my Hodgkin's, I resented going back to school and facing my old life, even if just for a few hours a day. I hated the idea that after all I had been through and after I had grown and learned so much, I was still the "nebech." I felt like screaming to all those clueless people out there, "I'm so happy to be who I am right now! I am miles ahead of you! My heart goes out to you that it will still take you years, if ever, to reach the point I stand at now."

I felt it was so ironic that I was the one who was so much more mature, but I was the odd one out.

Okay, to deflate my big head; I wasn't all that amazing. People like me never change their inner core, and in truth, I still was a monster. But I did feel that I had changed enough in certain areas and instead of being recognized for it, I was put down.

But that's enough rambling. I guess that's life. Not the life I expected after chemo, but life nonetheless.

Sunday, February 29, 2004

From Bald to Beautiful!

A week after "Remission Thursday," on a Friday, I went to get my sheitel done up for my cousin Leiba's wedding. I was so excited and couldn't stop directing the hairdresser and telling her exactly what I wanted my sheitel to look like.

I think she wanted to pin my mouth shut.

She kept looking at me strangely the entire time until she finally asked why kids like me got married so young. I debated telling her that my parents sold me off so that they could bring in the money to feed their other twenty-nine kids, but I finally settled on the cancer story because it sounded better.

I definitely made her feel bad. I felt like such a monster. In a good way though. Like a nice monster. Like Cookie Monster.

Sunday afternoon, Chai Lifeline made a Purim party. Faigy and I took the kids there because our parents were in Israel with Zevy to put on tefillin for the first time at our Rebbe's side.

Chavy and Eli went along with them as a sort of honeymoon reward for doing everything for us over the last few months. Chavy had also just told us that she was expecting, and she and Eli wanted to get some davening done while they were at the *kevarim* and *berachos* when they went to the rebbe.

We were so happy for her, but also so jealous that we weren't going along on that trip!

Zevy was the luckiest, because that trip was all about him, but all he could care about was that he was missing the Chai Lifeline party where they had free food, a Build a Bear Workshop, moonwalks, and all his favorite entertainers.

Silly boy. I would have switched places any day.

I begged Michal to come to the Chai Lifeline party and just say again that she was there because her father was a doctor. She didn't like the idea, but she did say she would meet me afterward and we'd go to the mall together. I was fine with that!

The hard part of the day was facing all the girls from our school who were there as volunteers for Chai Lifeline. We felt that it was a great organization that we associated with something very personal to us; my family's struggle to cope with my illness. It was always refreshing to meet other people at Chai Lifeline functions who were just like us, but meeting up with schoolmates who were there, not understanding what we were going through, but just there to complete *chesed* hours and to get accepted to work in Camp Simcha, was unnerving.

I brought my scrapbook along to show some of my Chai Lifeline friends, and it was a huge hit. I don't think anyone there had ever seen their illness from the point of view I put it in. I was really proud to show that around. It was great to be able to show people what I had been through but in a lighthearted, cheerful way.

After the party, Faigy and I got the kids to where they were staying while my parents were gone and met Michal at the bus stop next to the mall. We were having such a good time until Michal's sister sent a text to my phone that I should keep an eye on her because her white blood counts were low and she really wasn't supposed to be running around.

I didn't tell Michal anything, but I worried until we got her home.

In the mall we all went nuts trying on hats and funny shoes and Faigy messed around at the makeup counter and came back looking slightly strange. Michal had to help her get it all off, but some of it stayed on and Faigy looked a bit like a five-year-old that got caught in her mommy's makeup bag.

In Macy's we bumped into my friend Miri, who was surprised to see that I knew Michal. She knew Michal from her school and said that she was a top girl. I knew all that already, but Miri told me that Michal was tutoring some classmates of hers for the math regent and she had been *chagigah* head the year before.

I was suddenly very shy to be around Michal. She was so popular and so talented and so smart and also a year older than me. She was amazingly strong about her situation and I could never imagine doing everything she was.

Every new bit of information gave me a better idea of why Michal wanted to be so quiet about her ordeal. She was at the top of her school. She was the one helping everyone else. To go from where she was to becoming the object of everyone's pity was not something anyone wanted to do, least of all Michal.

Miri was dying to know how we knew each other, but Faigy saved the day by saying that Michal's father was the doctor I went to in case of an emergency when I couldn't get to Hackensack.

I think Michal could have hugged Faigy then.

Something really cheerful that was also happening at that time was the reappearance of my hair! It was soft and fuzzy and really dark! It was completely different from the reddish brown hair I had before chemo. You couldn't really see it yet, but you could feel my new hair if you closed your eyes and concentrated on wanting to feel the fuzz. Shmully and Nechama and Yitzy were always busy feeling my almost non-existent hair. No one else believed I had any, but the younger kids and I had good imaginations. We believed in magic!

I started taking pictures once a month to document my hair as it grew. I had this idea of putting a page in my scrapbook with a year's worth of pictures and calling it "From Bald to Beautiful."

Ayala and Miri dropped by Friday night to see my new fuzz. My hair was so short you couldn't see it unless it was under a very bright light, and even then it just looked like my head was dirty. But because I had been bragging about my new locks, they insisted on seeing my head. They made such a big fuss over what they didn't see. It was better than when Ayala had come to my house the last time and commented on my gorgeous new haircut before she figured out it was a sheitel.

My eyebrows had just started to fall out, but beneath the longer hairs that were coming out, shorter ones were already growing in. They were really light, but I was able to pencil them in for the few weeks it took until they grew in completely.

I was still pale and emaciated and my eyes were humongous because my cheeks were non-existent. No amount of makeup was able to make me look less frail. But I just looked so much better than I had looked a few short weeks before on chemo that I thought I looked awesome then.

I was so proud of being well again, that I was shocked one night later that week when I got a very rude reminder that in my community I'd never be considered perfectly normal again ....

Monday, March 01, 2004

Shira's Neshameleh

*M*onday was possibly the worst day I had since starting this journal.

Michal's sister called me early in the morning to tell me that Michal's friend Shira had passed away.

I never knew her friend, but I cried all morning and asked my mother if I could go to the *levayah*.

Michal was there right up with her friend's family, crying as if she was one of Shira's sisters. I sat in the back; I don't think Michal even knew I was there. I watched her the whole time, and I cried for her and davened that she should get well. I never wanted to lose her the way she lost her friend.

I watched from way in the back as Shira's family struggled

to follow along with the *Tehillim* being read. Shira had been becoming frum on her own and her family was slowly following. I never met Shira, but from what I saw after she passed away, I knew she must have been an amazing person.

Michal fainted when she stood to walk behind the *aron*, and I lost sight of her as her father and some Hatzoloh members crowded around to make sure she was fine.

I couldn't stay any longer and left.

I spoke to Michal's sister over the phone that night to find out when would be a good time to go see Michal, who insisted on staying with Shira's family while they were sitting *shivah*. She said that Michal kept fainting throughout the day, but refused to go into the hospital, so her father was staying with her the whole time.

I crawled into bed and stayed there most of the day, too upset to do anything more than cry and sleep and cry some more.

Michal and I spoke much later, but both of us were too drained to talk. We ended up just using up our cell phone minutes listening to each other breathe.

Michal gave me a beautiful letter she wrote during the *shivah*. I thought it was so touching, so I asked her if I could show it to others and she said it was okay as long as they didn't know she wrote it.

Here it is:

Shira dearest, *a"h*

I am sitting down now, trying to capture your essence on paper. You *can't* be written down on paper, though; you were much more dimensional than ink on paper can possibly be. Whatever I write here will not be doing you proper justice, yet it's something for me to hold onto.

I think the first aspect of your personality that struck me was your smile. From before I was diagnosed, your sweet, encouraging smile was there, inviting me to bask in your glow. It wasn't just a beautiful smile, but it reflected and expressed your genuine personality. You exuded an outgoing warmth and openness. It's as though it was yesterday, having been introduced to my illness, feeling as though I was transported to a strange, new planet. You saw me, became my friend, and I became yours. You welcomed me to the hospital, knew what to say, when to just sit, and when to go. You also coached and helped me navigate through the technical mazes of cancer treatments, doctors, tests, and checkups. Daily checkups are frightening and unnerving, but I always relied on meeting you, and we'd end up laughing together. You taught me that it's okay to laugh at things that aren't laughing matters. We discussed how we might be "finished" and expected to return to normal. But then we realized that "normal" is relative, and that things will never return to the way they were. You giggled and said, "Thank goodness!"

Another window to your unique *neshamah* were your eyes. Deep green, they exuded your search for *emes*. There are few people like you, faced with an ordeal like yours, who simultaneously took it as a stepping stone to reach greater heights. I remember vividly the times we spent schmoozing together, when I'd space out, just staring into your eyes. They said it all. Your eyes were so sensitive and soft, determined and dancing. I always told you — you don't have to say a word — your eyes give it all away. So many facets of yourself were there to be read in your eyes — I can't possibly forget them.

For the duration of our relationship you had no hair, but you had a magnificent crown on your head. I always marvel at your refined dignity that you possessed through the very end. When we spoke for the first time after you relapsed, I may have thought I'd have to encourage you. Of course, you encouraged me, and apologized for making me feel shaky about my own health. You apologized, Shira! I don't know anyone with your strength.

You expressed yourself so well through song. Hearing you hum was quite common. There are many songs that now have your stamp on them in my mind. It was already close to your *petirah*, at the height of your pain, when you sang Abie Rotenberg's "*Neshamale*" to me on the phone. I cried then, and I'm crying now. I don't think I'll ever be able to hear that song again without feeling choked up inside. But your songs evoke happy memories, too. I recall you sitting alongside me, after one of my surgeries, both of us in wheelchairs. You were whispering, talking almost more to yourself than to me, about how life is really a song. There are altos and sopranos, highs and lows, harmonies, and chords played. Certain parts alone may sound ugly, but in synchronized perfection, the music is bliss. Your orchestra resounded with perfection, Shira, and you lived your life with bliss.

Shira, I know you're in a better place now. Still, I miss you so much! I have so much to tell you, and I need you to talk to me! I need to hear your soothing voice, saying it's okay. You assured me that we'd both push double-carriages together. You're so close to Hashem now, even closer than you were before. Beg Him, please, for all of *Klal Yisrael*, and for me. We all need your *tefillos* so much — don't stop until *Mashiach* comes.

I'll be looking out for you in Yerushalayim any day now.

T'hei nishmasaich tzrurah b'tzror hachaim.

I love you so much,
Michal

Tuesday, March 02, 2004

She's BALD under That Thing!!!

*T*wo days before Leiba's wedding was five days before Purim, and my mother needed something from the grocery that night. She sent me to a supermarket a few blocks away and I went over in my bandanna. It was nine at night and I didn't want to get dressed just to pick up a bottle of milk. I figured I could leave my house and be back within ten minutes.

I was wrong. It was *erev* Purim and the store was mobbed. Everyone was doing their last-minute shopping for *mishloach manos*, and it took me ten minutes just to get to where they kept the milk.

I got a lot of stares as I was navigating my way through the crowds, but I just blushed and ignored most of them. There were some kids who pointed fingers, but I pretended not to notice when their mothers told them to shush.

As I got in the line to pay, a young married woman, not that much older than I was, stopped me. She was wearing some ratty old housecoat and a *tichel* and she had the nerve to tell me, "I don't know where you are from, but here we don't dress this way."

I felt like I had just been slapped. I turned to her and said, "It happens to be that you are lucky I'm from this community because you are setting a pretty poor example for what the people here are like. If I didn't live a few blocks away, I would probably think that all people from this place were as judgmental as you are."

The lady looked really angry when I said that and told me she wished she knew my name because she wanted to tell my school what a *chilul Hashem* I was making by coming out in a bandanna.

I recited my *Tehillim* name and told her that if she kept me in mind when she davened sometime it would be like a *chesed* for the day.

You were able to hear the *entire* store take a collective gasp. The cashiers were not doing anything, the lines weren't moving. Everyone was busy watching our confrontation.

I went on to tell her that it did not take much of a brain to figure out why I was bald and I didn't think it took that much common sense to keep quiet about it. Instead of apologizing, or at least keeping quiet, she still had the nerve to tell me that even if I were sick, I still had to be responsible and make sure to look good when I went out. I had to get myself a nice sheitel because otherwise people would stare.

I couldn't believe her chutzpah, so I countered with some of my own and asked her if she wanted to pay for that sheitel.

She said there were plenty of cheap synthetics out there.

I fought back and said, "Look, I'm a sixteen-year-old kid. You think there is a single person in the frum community who will not recognize a sheitel when they see one? What sixteen-year-old kid wants to be pointed at? If I'm going to get a wig, it had better be the most amazing and natural-looking one on the market so that NO ONE is going to be able to tell that it's not my hair. Unfortunately there is no such thing as a sheitel not being recognized anymore in the frum world, and people like me don't spend that kind of money on those amazing sheitlach anyway.

"Instead, I am very comfortable with what I look like and what I am going through, and I am not shy to walk out and be myself no matter what anyone thinks. They are pointing at me anyway. Let them point and say, 'I admire her guts,' instead of, 'Poor kid who has to wear a sheitel.'"

The woman still didn't know when to stop. She called me on the fact that I was exposing the community's kids to something they didn't need to see.

Oh, that got me so angry!

I asked her why it was okay for kids to daven for me when I was in the hospital but when I was well enough to walk around, they should not be exposed to the likes of my bald head. If anything, frum kids should be coming to visit people like me in the ward so that they'd grow up with an understanding of what they were davening for instead of being repulsed and afraid of a sick child.

And then I wanted to know why it was that now, when I was finally well enough to be a normal daughter again, and run errands for my mother at such a hectic time, my bandanna was the problem.

You could have heard a pin drop. I'd had enough of talking, so I just walked past everyone standing in line before me, dumped my bottle of milk on the counter, paid, and walked out.

As I reached the door, I turned back to that poor, delusional lady, and told her, "Before you make a comment like this again, get your priorities straight. And by the way, thanks for all your support."

Then I walked home and completely put the matter out of my head. I couldn't help it if people wanted to be stupid. I didn't even tell my parents. As it turned out, they told me.

Thursday, march 04, 2004

We've Got Cancer in Common ... Let's Get Married!

*T*he next day, I went to school with a baseball cap on top of my sheitel even though some teachers commented that they didn't like when I did that.

Feeling so self-assured because of last night's incident in the grocery store, I brought a bandanna along in my backpack, just in case. I figured that I was going to just take the whole sheitel off and put on my bandanna if anyone made a single comment to me again.

Thankfully, no one commented, but at the end of the day it started pouring as we were leaving the school building. Without thinking, I slipped off my sheitel and put the bandanna on instead and walked home with my wig in my bag.

The teacher who had been quite nasty to me about the cap stood there and stared with her mouth open as my friends all walked me home.

Felt good!

Thursday was Taanis Esther and that night was Leiba's wedding. I was so excited to finally feel good enough to dress up again and go out looking nice. I spent the entire day looking at my gown and doing my makeup over ten times and then finally going over and getting Leiba's makeup artist to do it for me, and then doing it myself again.

I thought I looked amazing at Leiba's wedding, but when I looked back at pictures I realized that as good I looked, I still had a long way to go before looking completely healthy.

In the middle of the dancing, someone told me that my father was looking for me at the *mechitzah*, so I went over to see what he wanted. I was a little annoyed when he introduced me to my brother-in-law's friend, a boy named Shlomo who was also sick with Hodgkin's. He left us to talk about what we had in common.

I felt so stupid. We cancer survivors aren't always on the lookout to meet other survivors and talk about chemo. We like to live normal lives and talking about chemo is tiresome and not what we're about.

I think people thought that two chemo patients must always be meant for each other because they have something so major in common.

I really didn't think chemo could be a common denominator in a relationship. I felt that the relationship could be a lot stronger if based on what we both *got* and *learned* from our experiences rather than the experience itself. Two people don't have to go through the same rough ride in order to make them right for each other. What makes them suited to each other are the similar perspectives on what they have gone through individually.

It was fine talking to Shlomo, but I walked away feeling he was "just another kid with cancer." I had nothing in common with him. I think my father was slightly disappointed that I didn't want to marry him on the spot.

I hoped that when it came time for me to look for my *basherte*, people would be understanding of the person I was despite the "damages" inflicted upon my resume because of the cancer. I thought I had a lot to offer because of what I had gone through, and I was worried that I wasn't going to be given the chance to be a normal kid because the people around me didn't see me that way.

It hurt to think of all the people out there who must be having such a hard time finding their *basherte* because they were being stereotyped. Cancer patients are the same as mental patients for all the people around me seemed to care or know or care to know.

I was still too young to be overly concerned with this issue, but I always wondered how people dealt with it.

Meeting Shlomo really made me think hard about it, and then later when Yossi asked what we had spoken about, I had to wonder about him. What was life like for him? He was a divorcé who wasn't getting set up with anyone half-decent. Being divorced meant that his marriage wasn't *basherte* to last, it didn't mean he was a bad person who deserved to be a second-class candidate for marriage.

I was shy to ask him about it, but I was sure it was an issue for him. There had been so many times where he had said he didn't believe he deserved half the problem cases he was set up with. He said that he felt like a regular guy and he wanted to be considered one.

I'm not sure if I understood him because he made sense, or just because I was in the same situation. When I spoke to people about this issue, many agreed with me, but still would never take that step and go out with someone they didn't think was in their league of "perfect people."

Then there were others who insisted I didn't see the other side of things. Someone I once spoke to said she would never trust anyone who had an "interesting" background because people tend to lie about medical conditions and such. I heard what she was saying, but then again, people lie all the time when it comes to *shidduchim*. How many stories did I know about couples who were *top* kids and then after they got married all the secrets started to come out?

I knew there wasn't any right or wrong way to approach this issue, and that I was going to have to deal with it when my time came in the best way for me. But that night, even at sixteen, I felt indignant, maybe a little hurt, and also a bit sorry for myself.

Sunday,
March 06, 2004

You Scream for Ice Cream

Over Shabbos I heard that there were some pictures being passed around of me talking to Shlomo at Leiba's wedding. Some men who had been watching us talk had snapped pictures just so they could say that they had photos of us together even before we got married. As if it were a given I was going to marry Shlomo one day.

I hate those people who think they know everything and usually know it all at your expense.

Motza'ei Shabbos was Purim and we had to rush to shul as soon as Shabbos was over to hear the Megillah. I could have gone to a later reading, but I wanted to be home to help my mother clean up and set up whatever we needed for our *seudah* guests and everything. Faigy agreed to babysit while we were out and she went to the later reading with Leah Freund.

My family would not know how to do Purim without me. Every year I get all into it and come up with a theme and pretty much force everyone to wear identical costumes. I also write a poem of the entire Megillah story and tie in words that have to do with the theme.

That year a *cholov Yisrael* Carvel ice-cream shop had opened in the neighborhood and I came up with the idea of dressing up as Carvel employees. We had the whole getup. All nine of us plus Chavy and Eli and my parents wore black shirts with white aprons and white caps. The aprons and caps had the Carvel logo ironed on to them.

My mother and Ruchie and I all wore our costumes to shul and we brought along my father's and the ones for Zevy and Pinny and Dovid and Shmully.

After the Megillah reading was over, I ran to where my father and Ruchie and my mother were all standing waiting for me. Yossi was schmoozing with my father and I heard him say that his parents weren't home for Purim so he was jumping around for the meal.

Of course my mother invited him over, and he said only if we carried pistachio ice cream.

My mother actually went and bought a tub of pistachio on the way home that night. I was so nauseated. Who still eats pistachio ice cream? Yuck.

I wasn't wearing a sheitel when Yossi came into my house later, only a baseball cap. My father wasn't happy when I took it off to let Nechama feel my fuzzy-wuzzy head. He said that since I was in remission I had to stop focusing on my having been sick and I needed to start wearing a sheitel and looking good and being a regular teen again.

I have no idea what that was supposed to mean. How regular a teen can one be while bald?

My father and Zevy were excitedly showing Yossi around our recently remodeled basement when a whole group of *bochurim* came dancing through our front door. My father isn't into these things because we try to put the little ones to bed as soon as possible so that we can get an early start in the morning.

Yossi ran up from the basement and apologized to the boys but said his father-in-law wasn't home. The *bochurim* laughed and said that they weren't dancing for money, they were sent by an organization to dance for me because I was sick.

So much for being normal again.

I told my father I should have stayed in my bandanna because so many people were coming and expecting to cheer up a sick girl, and they were all disappointed to find me looking so well.

Sunday, March 07, 2004

WE All Scream for Ice Cream!

I had a full day on Purim. My family always does.

We wake up really early every year and start making our *mishloach manos* rounds before most people are even home from shul. Chalk it up to my mother; she has her routes planned by Sukkos time and the alternate back up plans finalized by Chanukah.

The girls pile into one car and my father takes the boys in the other. By two in the afternoon we are always done and back at the house.

I had been off chemo for a little over a month now, but I was still extremely weak. It actually took over a year before I was physically back to myself. An entire day of Purim was more than enough to really wipe me out. By the time the meal came around, I was in a bandanna sleeping on the couch. I was exhausted at the thought of eating or even of looking at more food. Even though we had tons of people walking through our front door, no one said anything about my army-fatigue-print kerchief. I don't think the bandanna really bothered anyone except my father.

I was just considering going up to my room when Yossi walked in. Of course, my father asked me to go put on my sheitel. I told him I would have loved to accommodate him, but my hair was in use by Pinny, who was dressing as a Carvel waitress. My father said I was more than welcome to embarrass myself.

As if interesting situations ever bothered me before!

My brother commented on Yossi's funny cap and said it was so sweet that an old man like him made the effort to get dressed up for Purim. Yossi blushed and said it was a hat that he wore all the time.

Talk about embarrassing!

It happened to be a regular peaked cap and there was nothing strange about it at all, but I had never seen anyone his age wear something like that unless he was born in Switzerland or Austria or one of those other European countries.

He traded his cap for my brother's Carvel apron, and he again was part of the family. He even offered to help serve during the meal. My brothers tried to get him drunk, and the more he drank the more we laughed. He didn't seem so old when he told my brother Shmully that he liked Uncle Moishy tapes more than Shmully did.

My grandmother joined me on the couch and asked me what I was planning to do about school and I told her about my dilemma. I explained how I felt I was so mature now and that I was way past all that high-school stuff.

Yossi overheard and asked me why I didn't finish up my last few Regents and then decide what I wanted to do. If I had my diploma in hand I could leave any time I wanted to.

It wasn't such a bad idea coming from someone who had all that to drink.

Of course he couldn't resist the ultimate tease by telling me to just get married. He sounded just like when my father used to tell me to cut off my head to get rid of a pimple.

My father joined us on the couch later, and noticing my bandanna, he told us about this crazy story he heard about a girl who had stopped an entire grocery store defending her bald head. He was admiring her nerve as I turned red and tried to bury myself in the carpet. He was saying how everyone in shul was talking about it and kept asking him if it was his kid who made the whole commotion.

He told everyone that his daughter did not have that much chutzpah.

My Uncle Shimi gave my father a funny look and said he heard the same story and that he heard that it *was* his kid doing all that.

Suddenly everyone noticed me and I had to tell them all what happened that night at the supermarket. All of a sudden I wasn't the girl with the nerve; I was the girl who was totally embarrassing to have as a daughter.

I knew it was a good idea not to talk too much about what had happened. As soon as I got home from the grocery, I had about ten phone calls from people who had already heard about a kid with a bandanna who made a scene, and they knew that it had to be me. I didn't think a small bald head could attract that much attention. I guess a small head with a big mouth *can* do a lot.

Yossi brought the conversation back around to me going back to school and he told my father that the best thing would be to marry me off before I got into too much trouble.

My father absolutely beamed and said, "You're my kind of man!"

Grrrrr!

I invited all the guests at my parents' house to my *seudas hoda'ah* later that week. My cousin Leiba had said it was okay to make it during one of her *sheva berachos* and told me to invite whomever I wanted to.

Originally, my father asked our Rav if we should make my *seudas hoda'ah* right away or if we should wait five years, since cancer patients are considered officially cured after five years in remission. Our Rav said that we should do it as soon as possible otherwise there was a chance we would forget and it would never get done.

My parents asked him if it was okay to make it together with Zevy's bar mitzvah, because it was coming up in a few weeks, and the Rav said that they shouldn't mix two *simchahs* at one time. He said that it was okay to make it with Leiba's *sheva berachos*, though, because it wouldn't be mixing two *simchahs* in the same family.

Of course, my parents asked Leiba if she minded and not only did she not mind, she was very excited to be able to say yes.

Yossi promised he'd be there and asked me if I needed help making up my speech. He told me to call him or email him if I needed any writing tips. All my cousins laughed and told him that of all people I didn't need any help writing.

As my grandparents were leaving, my grandfather tried to give me Purim *gelt*, but I gave it back. I told him I was too old for it. He said I deserved a present just for getting well. I told him that in that case I deserved something much better than just twenty bucks.

He agreed.

I had a lot of fun that day, but I was maxed out. I fell into bed and started the countdown to regular life.

Tuesday, March 09, 2004

Seudas Hoda'ah

I was unsure of what to do all night at my *seudas hoda'ah*. I invited my classmates and friends, but it was weird to accept *mazal tovs* for something that wasn't a typical *simchah*. All I could think to do was smile and say hi to everyone and then blush when I didn't know what else to say.

Chavy assured me that this was the normal process for anyone who was the recipient of a mazal tov. She said it was good practice for my upcoming *simchahs, im yirtzah Hashem.*

So many people came to wish me well and I got emotional thinking of how many people really cared for me and were genuinely happy at the news of my remission.

My poems were in frames right at the entrance to the hall, and everyone who walked in took a look at them. It made me shy but it felt nice to know that people thought they were good.

I took lots of pictures that night and when they were developed a little while later I laughed at how I thought I had looked good at my *seudas hoda'ah*. My suit was too big, my face was pale, my skin was greenish, and I had really thin eyebrows. I knew that the *simchah* was not about how I looked, but about how I was feeling, and I felt better, happy, and relieved, now that it was all over.

Of course I was still nervous about getting back to things, but worrying wasn't for that night. March 9th was my night to focus on how great life was and how thankful I was to be there, a healthy person again.

My cancer scrapbook was making the rounds and my mother and I were thrilled with all the compliments. My friend even heard some of our teachers talking about getting me on board the yearbook staff the next year.

I was so happy.

I looked into the men's section and it was full too! Of course, most people were there for my cousin Leiba, but there were plenty who had come for me. Yossi wasn't there yet, but as I turned to go back to the women's side of the room, I saw him coming into the hall.

As he was going to grab a piece of cake, my school principal walked in together with his wife. Yossi and I went to greet them together. Yossi knew my principal because they had once spoken about a *shidduch*. They exchanged handshakes, and then my principal turned to wish me all the best. He said his mandatory *mazal tov* and then gave me a look and said that *im yirtzah Hashem* he hoped to be at my *vort* around two months from then.

I thought I would die blushing.

I reminded the principal that I was only sixteen, and he said it didn't matter. His wife was the same age when he married her.

Yikes.

I kept waiting for Michal to come, but I didn't see her. She had told me she was going to be the first one to give me *mazal tov*, but it was already late and she wasn't there. I got a little worried and left the hall for a few minutes to call her on her cell phone.

Before I even got to call her, I noticed that I had a missed call from Michal's home number. I listened to the message and it was from her sister, telling me that Michal wasn't going to make it that night. I called her sister back and she told me that Michal had some complications with a medicine she was taking and was rushed into the hospital. I asked for more details but her sister couldn't tell me anything else. She said she was waiting for details too.

She asked me that even though her family was keeping Michal's illness a secret, could I please have everyone at my *seudas hoda'ah* say some *Tehillim* for her?

I didn't know what to say after that, so I begged her to please let me know when she heard anything about Michal and I would for sure say some *Tehillim* for her.

I rushed to my mother as soon as I hung up the phone to tell her what I just heard. I was devastated. Of all people, Michal would have made my *simchah* complete that night. She understood where I was coming from, and was hoping to get to where I was. I worried about her all night and kept checking my phone for messages.

I asked my father to say some *Tehillim* out loud on the mike for all the people who were still sick and I gave him a list of names that I knew and added Michal's name to the bottom. I hoped that no one would know her name, because I didn't think Michal would ever forgive me for putting it out there in public.

I finally got a text message from Michal herself saying that she was fine but tired and was going to fill me in on the details later. I was still worried, but much calmer after that.

After that episode, it was time to give my speech. First, I thanked Chavy and Eli for giving so much of their time and strength to keep everything running smoothly while I was taking up all of my parents' energy. Then I thanked Faigy for giving up on being a normal teen for a while to take on the huge responsibility of keeping everything going while I was sick. I presented Faigy with a gold link bracelet that had a red *Kever Rochel* string threaded through each link. My parents had picked it up in Israel when they were there with Zevy and wanted me to give it to Faigy from all of us.

Then I read my "Train" poem, and made a lot of ladies cry and then I read something I wrote for my parents.

> *Have you ever looked up to wish upon a star?*
> *I know I have.*
> *Have you ever felt disappointed when at night, the stars don't appear?*
> *I know I have.*
> *And have you ever had a star or constellation that was special to you? One that you looked for and looked up to most?*
> *I know I do.*
> *Tatty and Mommy, you are two of those special stars in my life.*
> *Whether I see you there or not, I know that like a star, you are constant. You mean constant support, friendship, and love.*
> *I know that even when I don't see you, you're there anyway, like the stars that hide on a cloudy night.*

They all come out eventually, maybe another night, but they'll be there for me again and again and always and forever, I know they'll keep on shining.
Thank you so much Tatty and Mommy!

I think I made some people cry then too.

My Aunt Kayla and her daughter Chaya and all the other Rubinsteins got together to buy me a stunning white gold ring that had diamonds and sapphires set into it. I couldn't stop looking at it. It was the most beautiful piece of jewelry I had ever worn.

When I showed it to my father he said that I was making it very hard for any prospective *chasan* to impress me. He went around showing it off, saying that thing about a future *chasan*.

I did not find the whole situation funny.

When most of the guests had left the *sheva berachos* my father asked me to read my speech again in the men's section to the close friends who were still there. I was so shy; I barely looked up from my paper.

Zevy and Pinny were winking at me and made me laugh every time I did look up, and when my father noticed, he told everyone how silly I was for being shy when all these men had seen me bald and brought me food to the hospital when I was at my worst.

Oh, yay. Great end to a great night.

Wednesday, March 10, 2004

Back to School

I was still the sixteen-, almost seventeen-year-old me, not exactly the same as I had been four months before, but, I hoped, not that altogether different. True, I was missing that brick in my neck and some hair, but I was still the same kid with a sense of humor and a big mouth.

I tried to go back to school believing all that, but it was hard. I had changed a lot more than I thought I had.

I stopped writing in my Hodgkin's journal and hoped that cancer was behind me, but it seemed to want to follow me around everywhere. It wasn't so easy to forget.

I couldn't just pop back into school and blend in after being gone most of the year. I couldn't catch up with my school work and physically, I was not up to it and had to go home early most days.

I decided to study on my own and take my twelfth-grade Regents in June. Then I was going to take Yossi's advice and take it from there. I could go back to school and drop out later if I felt like it.

In the meantime, my friends had other friends, and I wasn't sure where I belonged and if I would ever really belong again.

I tried. But I think the social aspect was the hardest part of being sick. Chemo kills cancer. What kills loneliness?

Motza'ei Shabbos, March 13, 2004

NEVER Say NEVER

The Motza'ei Shabbos after my *seudas hoda'ah*, I decided that my hair was passable as a boy's, so I took one of Pinny's yarmulkes and paraded around the house. I was wearing one of his sweatshirts, too, so I guess I really did look like a boy.

Then the doorbell rang.

Forgetting what I looked like, I ran to open the door. It was one of my neighbors who came to ask my father something.

I told him *hi* and he looked at me strangely and asked, "Do I know you?"

Suddenly I realized that he didn't recognize me and thought I was a boy, and I blushed madly and told him I had no idea who he was either. I ran up to my room and changed quickly and even put on my sheitel before my father had to say anything.

Then I tried to disappear for the rest of the night.

The Landers made it easier on me by calling me over to babysit and it was a relief to get out. I can be lots of fun sometimes, but people don't always think my ideas are quite normal. I have to agree.

They came home pretty late and I was sure I was coming home to a sleeping house, but the lights were still on as I crossed the street. I walked into the living room just as Yossi Spitzer was leaving, carrying some more of my teddy bear presents. I was planning to donate them to the Hackensack playroom because lately I hadn't been able to find my bed due to the number of presents I had.

I later found out that the reason I couldn't find my bed was because my father took it down to the garage to make more room for all my teddy bears.

Yossi figured that if I wasn't going to use the bears, he had a little nephew that would love them. He showed me pictures of his little cutie and then had to leave to take another nephew of his out for pizza.

My father wanted to know why his little nephew was still up so late at night, and Yossi laughed and explained that he had nephews who were older than me. He was the youngest in his family and his oldest brother was even older than my father so he had nieces and nephews who were his age.

I couldn't imagine it. It turned out that one of his nieces had been my substitute in seventh grade! It was really weird.

When he finally left, I asked my parents why Yossi had been there for so long.

They looked at each other and said that he had been talking to them about a *shidduch* that came up and seemed very promising.

I was excited for him. I really was. He was an amazing person and I thought he deserved to be happy. I felt a little bad because my own future was so uncertain — I didn't even know if I was going back to school! And then *shidduchim* could be such a struggle after illness.

My parents asked if I had anything to say and I said that no one needed my opinions because I was not going to interfere with Yossi's life. I was happy for him and I thought the girl was very lucky to get a man like him and I hoped that one day when it was my turn I could find someone like that too.

My father then sat me down to have a little talk.

It seemed that for the past week there had been a lot going on behind my back. There was someone who called my father, trying to set Yossi up with me. My parents spoke to Yossi for a long time before they even wanted to tell me about it.

Yossi hadn't gone on any *shidduchim* since December because he had put every possibility on hold ever since he met me. He knew that I was much younger and that there was a huge chance that nothing was ever going to come out of waiting for me, but he wanted to stick around until I was old enough to think about it.

He didn't say anything to anyone about this, because he thought it would be inappropriate, but when someone randomly put him together with me, he told my parents what he really felt.

I was so shocked; I didn't know what to say. Not having something to say is a first for me.

I argued that I was so young, but my parents admitted that even though I wasn't going to be seventeen for a few months, I was already very mature.

I reminded them that they were calling the girl who had a stomachache named David *mature*, but they laughed and said that I was mature when it came to life experience. My personality was probably never going to change.

They had asked our Rebbe for advice and he said to leave it all up to me. If I thought I was ready, it was time for me to go on with my own life.

I said that I was flattered that Yossi wanted to date me seriously, but I was a little overwhelmed by all of it. I wasn't sure what to make of it all and I wanted time to think. It was all way too strange for me to get a grip on in one night. This was the sort of thing that happened in books, not in real life.

My life is always active; there's always something happening around me, but this was the cherry on top.

I always said that I would never marry someone with a shtreimel or someone named Spitzer, but it seems that now I was about to date both.

Monday, October 25, 2004

My Chai Lifeline Driver

*Y*ossi and I formally met shortly after that *Motza'ei Shabbos* and we were engaged on my seventeenth birthday. We met for a few months before making our engagement public even though we knew from the first time that we were going to live happily ever after.

We were waiting for a few things, one of them for my body to recover from chemo. There was a lot we didn't know about how my life would be after cancer, and we were giving it some time to get back to normal before making any big decisions for life.

Of course, I knew I was going to be fine, but still, I wished I was a few years ahead in time to actually see that for myself. I was worried a lot of the time that Yossi would have to wait forever for me to get back to myself, but he was always so sweet about it. He told me once that a rose takes a full year to bloom. If people could wait a year for a rose, he could wait for me too.

It was quite embarrassing to know that Yossi's parents and our Rebbe and the other people who were involved in our *shidduch* were all discussing the private issues I had with my health, but I didn't really have a choice. It was understandable. They all wanted the best for us and didn't want to make decisions without knowing everything there was to know first. I was very uncomfortable with it, but hey, cancer didn't ask permission to take over.

Because we weren't officially a *shidduch* until some issues were cleared up, Yossi found other ways to take me out. He used to drive me to Hackensack for my checkups or he would pick me up from school when I was too tired to stay a full day.

Once, a family at Hackensack noticed Yossi waiting for me in the waiting room and they asked me who he was. I didn't know what to say, so I told them he was my Chai Lifeline volunteer driver.

I'm a terrible liar, but the story made sense to them and Yossi and I laughed about it the whole way home.

We got engaged on my birthday, the day I turned seventeen. Seventeen sounds really young, and it is, but there's no such thing as a young person after cancer. I was still the same ball of fire and still the same terror when I wanted to be, but I had matured in other ways. My outlook and perspective on life were much deeper now. The people who knew me all understood how important it was for me to move on and not look back anymore.

My engagement was in my house, and it was just so full of people. I didn't know that our kitchen could hold so many guests! It was overwhelming to see how many people knew and cared and came for me. If I wasn't so worried about ruining my makeup, I would have cried.

It was so odd to hear some people saying, "Well if *you* can get engaged, it gives hope to all the other single girls out there!" What am I; the Abominable Snowman? I knew what they meant — they were trying to say that if a girl with cancer got engaged it was an inspiration to the others who were waiting to find their *basherte*, just because it typically is harder for a girl like me to find a *shidduch*. But whoa; the way it was phrased sounded really bad at first.

It did make me a little indignant, but I knew I had to let it go. I wasn't going to change the way the world thought of my illness, but I didn't have to let them get to me.

Of course, there were a lot of people from Hackensack at my engagement. To them it was such a *simchah* to see a cancer patient going on with life. I felt so special being able to give them *chizuk*.

Some of the women from Hackensack peeked into the men's section of the room to look at my *chasan* and suddenly began exclaiming about how I was marrying that Chai Lifeline guy they had met in the hospital.

Even today, when people hear my name they'll ask if I was the one who married that Chai Lifeline guy. I've even heard it from Chai Lifeline volunteers! I must apologize to Chai Lifeline about all that. The volunteers are wonderful people who are only looking to do *chesed*. They don't drive people to the hospital and then marry them. That was just the first thing that came to mind when I was asked who Yossi was.

My engagement was a little interesting because I was so young. My friends were still in high school while I was shopping for linen and pots and furniture. It was hard on me, but my real friends were always there. They were so good about keeping up our friendship even though it wasn't easy when I was sick and then engaged and living a completely different life than they were.

Miss Riegler (who was now Mrs. Glick) was also great. She knew the ropes when it came to an engagement and made shopping for towels and bathroom sets fun.

When it came to the day of my wedding, I was told to choose a *kabbalah* for the rest of my life that would always remind me of the *kedushah* of my wedding day. What came to mind was the time when my mother cried because she wasn't dressed for Shabbos as she lit the candles in my hospital room. Even though I knew I would always be dressed by the time I lit candles, I knew that whenever I *bentched licht*, I would remember a lot more than just the *kedushah* of my *yom chupah*. I knew that I would remember how special it was to celebrate Shabbos healthy and in my own home and not in some hospital bed craving hemoglobin.

Our wedding was just about a year to the day I found that brick in my neck. It was like another *seudas hoda'ah* for me to dance that night with all the people who cared for me and helped me over the last year.

Our wedding date was October 25, and in Hebrew it was *Yud Cheshvan*. *Yud Cheshvan* was the night, a full year ago, that my Aunt Carla and my cousin with the same name had that dream about my grandfather and his brother dressed to go somewhere special.

I walked down to the *chupah* to the tune of Yaakov Shwekey's "Mama Rochel." Because my *chupah* was after night fell, it was already *Yud Aleph Cheshvan*, Rochel Imeinu's yahrtzeit. I felt that it was so appropriate to walk down to her memory.

I thought of my sisters Chavy and Faigy and how much they did for me over the last year, just like Rochel Imeinu did for her sister, and of course I thought of my mother, who was holding my hand as she was leading me to my next stage in life, and how she cried for me and brought me to this place, just as Mama Rochel was doing in *Shamayim*.

It struck me a little later that the song "Mama Rochel" fit my typical Jewish song requirements. It encompasses marriage, family, and G-d.

I invited Dr. Harris to have a *berachah* under my *chupah* but as much as he wanted to be there, he had a sick nephew who needed him in Israel. We did send him a wedding picture and I got to accept his personal *mazal tov* the next time Yossi took me for a checkup — this time as my husband.

I originally wanted a small wedding, just close personal friends and family. I always hated those weddings where there were so many people, it was possible to spend a whole night there and not know who the *kallah* was. I really wanted every-one there to be a part of my *simchah* and not have to feel like they were just one of the crowd.

I was shocked at how many close personal friends and family I had! My wedding was full of people who meant so much to me, and I tried to greet and dance with every single one of them. There were lots of girls who came out of curiosity; after all, I was getting married while they were still in high school, but I know that most of them were there for me.

Michal was announced in remission a week before my wedding, and she joined my *simchah* looking very frail, but so happy. I had a special dance just with her, and we both cried and laughed right in the middle of the dance floor and nobody knew why. But it didn't matter. We knew.

Whenever I look back at my wedding video I'm amazed all over again at how many people were there. I looked healthy and felt great and was happier than I had ever been.

Looking at those pictures you can just see that I plan to live happily ever after.

Almost Five Years Later

Today

Just about three years after I was done with chemo, we experienced another miracle when our son JB was born. We call him JB because when he was born he was so tiny, he looked like a jellybean. The nurses said that even Jellybean was too long for such a tiny little kid, so it was shortened to JB.

He's what my friends call the miracle baby. When I was in Hackensack I never imagined that cancer was going to lead me to meet Yossi and that one day we would have a precious baby of our own to love and care for.

I remember when I was feeling so down and Dr. Harris told me the *mashal* of a train going through tunnels. He told me that while I was on chemo I needed to turn around in my seat and see the light of the tunnel opening behind me; the opening from which I had come in from.

Then there were times where I didn't see any light at all, and Dr. Harris said that I needed to still trust that my train was going in the right direction because Hashem was the one guiding it.

Today I know that Dr. Harris was so right. I wrote his *mashal* into a poem even before I knew that Yossi and JB were going to be the light at the end of my tunnel. Now that I know all that, I still wouldn't change that poem. I think that the point was to trust Hashem no matter what I thought I saw or knew on my own.

Sometimes when I read my old diary I can't believe that I was the one who said all those rude things to her teachers and her doctors and the one who gave her headaches names.

But then again, when I think that I call my son *Jellybean*, I guess I haven't changed all that much.

I still have a box sitting at the top of my closet that is full of every card, hospital bracelet, photograph, and helium balloon that I had from the time when I was sick. I take it down sometimes when I'm cleaning and stop what I'm doing to go through it all. It brings back so many memories.

Yossi also had a box with him as we set up our home together. I don't know where he put his or if he still has it, but I know that everyone has a box of some sort. It doesn't matter what's in it, or if the box lies in a closet or in your heart. Mine is a Hodgkin's box, but other people's boxes are just as important, no matter what the label on it reads.

My cancer scrapbook still makes the rounds; I love showing it off to the newly diagnosed patients to show them what to expect and to tell them that one day they'll be sitting in my place showing others that there is light at the end of the tunnel.

This year Chanukah will be five years since Yossi and I met, and it will also mark my five years off chemo. This Chanukah I'm going to be considered in complete remission; cured. It seems unreal.

Every person has their own miracle ride; this is only mine.

Cancer does not define me, but it is a big part of who I am. Any life experience will help mold a person and cancer has definitely done that to me. I am proud to stand on the other side and be able to say that there is a life after cancer.

Some people claim that life can't ever be the same after an illness and they are right.

Life is never the same, it only becomes more special.

Afterword

In memory of "Michal bas Yaakov Moshe"

*In memory of my dear friend "Shira,"
who taught me what life is all about."*

I remember a deep conversation I once had with a close friend while I was going through chemotherapy. The crux of the discussion was about lessons I had learned from my ordeal, how it had changed me as a person and in my perspective on life. My friend expressed, with a twinge of jealousy, how she wished that she too would be presented with an opportunity for growth like the one I was being faced with.

Although I couldn't understand why she would voluntarily subject herself to numerous surgeries, chemotherapy, radiation treatments and all they entail, I was cognizant of the privilege I had to attain higher heights through my experiences.

Later in the day, when I had rethought the conversation (and when some medication had worn off, leaving me less woozy), I was disappointed with the lingering thought my friend brought up; that only those with life-death *nisyonos* have opportunity to grow.

The ultimate level, I felt, was to be able to take the regular, typical ins and outs of life, and find the stepping stones to growth within them.

Take davening for example. When I was sick, I knew I had no one to turn to but Hashem. Top doctors gave up on me; statistics doomed me to sure death. Of course I forged that connection with Hashem! The potency of *tefillah*, however, is not reserved for cancer patients! Anyone can have that relationship with Hashem; we are all His children.

I also know my perception of Hashem's presence in my life should not be limited to myself alone. When I was able to perceive the "*bashert*" behind situations; for instance, when I had surgery over Pesach vacation, and I didn't have to miss any school, I knew it was Hashem orchestrating my life for me. However, cancer is not the only thing Hashem orchestrates. We can come to the same realization when a *shidduch* is made, when a high school senior gets a coveted twelfth-grade position or acceptance to the "right" seminary, or when you find the parking space on Thirteenth Avenue. His Presence is not reserved for the cancer ward alone.

I have also attained a heightened sensitivity to other people and their life situations. Because of the manner in which I dealt with my illness, by keeping it quiet, I could better understand others who had real-life issues under wraps too. I felt with the girl whose parents were divorcing, with the teacher married for ten years without children, and with the friend whose brother is "at risk." It doesn't have to "take one to know one." With just a tad of placing oneself into another's shoes, anyone can relate to others with sensitivity.

When people tell me, "You're amazing," I tell them how I'm not, how growth in my situation was natural. Cancer is like those rock-climbing walls. I was forced to climb higher, to reach new heights, because the only other option would be to slide down and succumb to the pain and fear.

When I talk to girls who are feeling "unfulfilled" and "empty" because their lives are *baruch Hashem* so normal, I feel so bad for them. Not because they're "missing out" on cancer; I'm happy they're being spared what I experienced. I feel bad for them because they are denying themselves the opportunity to become fantastic individuals. They don't realize that the rocky wall is still in front of them and giving them the chance to climb up. In a situation like mine I had no choice but to reach higher, but imagine how special it is when people who were never forced to do so take the initiative and pull themselves to the top. We all have the opportunity, with different circumstances. It's not about the circumstances, it's about the will and desire.

All the best,
"Michal"

Acknowledgments
by "Tzipi"

*M*ost authors put their acknowledgements at the beginning of their books, but from my own experiences, no one reads them. I found that once the author has made an impression on the reader, the reader will be more likely to want to hear what the author has to say and read about whom she wants to thank.

The people I feel I need to mention are people who popped up all over my diary, and now that my readers are already familiar with these characters, I can thank them and know that whoever reads this will understand why the following individuals deserve my appreciation. I hope that some of you will actually read this part instead of skipping it as usual.

... And if my acknowledgements are treated in the same way as they would be if they were written at the start of my book, then I did not gain anything but didn't lose either.

The previous pages, my book, told the story of the journey I took through the dark tunnels of illness and recovery. As I typed the diary I kept during that trying time, I looked forward to seeing it in print. To me, the completion of this manuscript symbolizes the completion of a journey, a train ride I took through a dark spot in my life.

Yet, as I come closer to the finishing stages of this project, I have begun to realize that this was not a ride I took alone. I always knew there were other passengers riding the tracks with me, and now their faces come into even better focus.

My parents would claim that all the help, care, and guidance they provided were a given, something that any parent would have done. They can claim all they want, but I know that my parents have given me so much more than they ever imagined they did. Aside from the support and care they showed me always, it was, and still is, the amazing attitude they have on life that helped me take my challenges when they came and as they still come.

There is no way a child can ever express enough admiration and thanks to a parent, but I do want to show my gratitude and appreciation for them here. Thank you for everything Tatty and Mommy.

My sister Blimi deserves an entire paragraph all to herself for the mesiras nefesh she endured, taking care of the family while our parents were busy with me. My sister took a year out of her everyday life for my benefit, and there is no way I can thank her enough for making it easier on all of us. I'm sorry for poking fun at you in the book, but hey, that's what sisters do!

"You can't pick your sisters but you can pick your friends," *it's an old cliché, but it works. I have to say that my sister Blimi is my sister, my friend, and a part of who I am.*

To the rest of my siblings, who had to put up with a messed-up schedule, missing parents, some scary moments, and jealousy over my presents, thank you for being the best bunch of sisters and brothers out there! Who else could have turned my balding head into a comedy of an upsherin, and have helped me appreciate the softness of my fuzzy-wuzzy scalp? Thank you for the favors, the laughs, the tears, and all the joy.

One thing I can't resist ... Mwhahahah! You know I love you all.

Bruchy, you are the sister I actually was able to choose. I know you longer than I know anyone, and I know you deserve to be in here, but I can't begin to list for what. Even though you were not mentioned much in the book, you've been like a part of my family and so I must thank you for sticking by us and helping out as if you lived in my house instead of next door. I am just as happy as your real sisters are to wish you mazal tov and to welcome your husband into our family.

Of course, my story would not be complete without its happy ending, and so I must thank my in-laws who looked past my illness and accepted me, for who I am, as a person. Thank you for the encouragement, reviewing my manuscript dozens of times, and for all the advice and support.

And to my sisters-in-law and nieces, thanks for being the best audience! You brainstormed and corrected and criticized and praised my work and I am proud to hand you a finished product. Tzipi Caton thanks you very much! Your mark is all over this work even if your names aren't.

To the friends who stuck with me throughout everything. I owe you so much. Bracha, Soshi, Devoiry, and everyone else who knows they belong here; you helped me as only friends like you can. You never got sick of me being sick and kept our friendships strong even when I was too weak to do so. Thank you for being there and for still remaining a part of my life.

Mrs. Bechhofer!!! What would I have done without you? Thanks for all the kvetch rants and the collaboration on lesson plans and tests ... and of course, with your input on this book. I am so thankful for the way we met and that we got to know each other as well as we do. Without the experiences of Michal my book would be flat. I am so happy you agreed to share her story and thereby add dimension to mine. Because I really dislike advanced math, when you suggested a FOIL character, I wanted to disown you. I'm glad I didn't!

I can't write an acknowledgements page without mentioning all the wonderful people who helped my family during my illness. I tried to do some of you justice in the book, but there is no way. When it comes down to writing acknowledgements, and I have to begin choosing whom to mention and whom to leave out, it becomes extremely difficult. Everyone deserves to be recognized for everything they have done for us, but, as my mother mentioned in her foreword, there is no way to possibly list you all. But I still feel that credit is due, even in such a small paragraph. The babysitting, rides, food, suppers, Tehillim, and everything else you did for us to help make our burden easier really took a load off our hearts and minds. A dark tunnel can become a lot brighter with even a small dot of light. You were the glowing dots that helped us remember there was a light at the end of the tunnel.

To ArtScroll and Miriam Zakon, who have made my dreams a reality; you worked so quickly and impressed me with the quality in everything you did, and in how nice you all are! Accomplishing a goal is a little scary. It's something you hope for and never believe until it becomes real. Thank you for being the kind of people I had no doubts about trusting my hopes with. You handled them as carefully as if these were your own dreams, your own story going out to print, and took it all the way.

There are no words to convey what I wish to say about the man to whom I owe my recovery and my life. Dr. Michael Harris was the man who introduced me to the mashal of the train and sat with me to explain all the stops we took along the way. I thank him for being the shaliach who did so much more than care for my body; he encouraged my spirit at every turn.

Dr. Harris, please accept the thanks I can manage to give in these few lines, and know there is so much more that I find hard to express. Yes, it's shocking, but for once, "Glucose" is at a loss for words.

My husband always says he doesn't have to read my book because he lived it all with me, and he is right. His support and pride in my work are the reasons I kept writing and even rewriting it all when my hard drive crashed. You helped me when I was sick and since then have always been at my side. Thank you for everything and more.

My baby doesn't even know that I am thanking him here, but I want my readers to know that my child is the miracle that makes my story complete. He is truly the broad daylight at the end of my tunnel and is proof that there are always good things that come out of the dark times. He is too young to understand how much he means to us, and yet, I still want to show my gratitude for having him in my life. May he bring us only nachas.

Without Hashem Yisbroach guiding me in everything I went through and did, there would be nothing. So many times throughout my illness it was so brilliantly clear that He was there, showing us the way. Even the times when it was hard to see His hand, I was taught to trust the One driving the train, because, after all, He's the One calling all the stops.

I thank Hashem for causing the train of my life to take the stops that it did and I hope that the emunah I picked up along the way will last for all the other stops and tunnels I ever have to take in my life.

"Tzipi Caton"

Glossary

Ahavas Hashem: Love of G-d

aron: coffin

ayin hara: evil eye

bashert: destined

basherte: destined spouse

berachah, (pl.) *berachos*: blessing(s)

bikur cholim: visiting the sick

bitachon: faith

bochurim: unmarried young men

chasan: groom

chesed: act of kindness

chilul Hashem: desecration of G-d's Name

chizuk: encouragement (lit: strength)

choleh: sick person

cholov Yisrael: milk whose production was supervised by a Jew

choshuv: VIP (lit: important)

chupah: wedding canopy

daven, davening: pray(ing)

dayan: Rabbinic judge

d'var Torah: short speech on Torah topics

emes: Truth

frum: observant

gashmiyus: pertaining to the physical world

gelt (Yiddish): money

hachnasas kallah: the mitzvah of providing financial assistance for needy brides

halachah (pl): *halachos*: Torah law(s)

Hashem: G-d (lit: The Name)

Hashgachah pratis: Divine Providence

Hatzoloh: Worldwide Jewish volunteer ambulance and emergency services organization (lit: Rescue)

im yirtzah Hashem: if G-d desires

gemach: Free-loan or other free lending association

kabalah: binding resolution

Kaddish: Prayer recited by mourners

kallah: bride

kamiyah: amulet

kedushah: holiness

kever, (pl): *kevarim*: grave(s)

Kever Rochel: Rochel's Tomb

Klal Yisrael: the Jewish People

leining: the public reading of the Torah during prayer services

levayah: funeral

levayas hameis: (lit: escorting the deceased); to bring a Jew to burial

levush: clothing

licht bentchen: candlelighting

matzeivah: headstone

mechaneches: educator

mechatunim: in-laws

mechitzah: partition

minyan: quorum of ten men

mishebeirach: prayer said during Torah reading, usually for *the sick*

mishloach manos: gifts of food given on the Purim holiday

mitzvah, (pl) *mitzvos*: commandment(s)

morah: teacher

Motza'ei Shabbos: Saturday night, after the Sabbath

neshamah (diminutive: *neshamaleh*): soul

niftar: (n.) the deceased (v.) passed away

nisyonos: tests; ordeals

petirah: death

peyos: sidelocks

refuah (pl) *refuos*: cure(s)

refuah sheleimah: get well soon; complete cure

semichah: Rabbinic ordination

seudah: a meal, usually festive

Seudas Hoda'ah: Meal of Thanksgiving

Shabbos: Sabbath

shadchan, (pl) *shadchanim*: matchmaker(s)

Shalosh seudos: third Sabbath meal

Shamayim: Heaven

shanah rishonah: first year of marriage

sheitel: wig

sheitelmacher: wig stylist

Sheva berachos: The festive meals honoring bride and groom during the week after their wedding

shidduch, (pl) *shidduchim*: match(es)

shiur: Torah class

shivah (sitting shivah): Week of mourning for the deceased

shtreimel: fur-trimmed hat worn by certain chassidic groups

siddur, (pl) *siddurim*: prayer book(s)

simchah: joy; joyous event

tefillah, (pl) *tefilos*: prayer(s)

Tefillas HaShachar: morning prayers

Tehillim: Psalms

tichel: headscarf

tzadekes: saintly woman

tzniyus: modesty

upsherin (Yiddish): first haircut, given to a boy at the age of three

vort: engagement party

yahrzeit: anniversary of a death

"*yene machlah*" (Yiddish): "that disease" (i.e., cancer)

yeshuos: salvation

yom tov: holiday

zechus: merit

zivug, (pl) *zivugim*: destined spouse(s)

z'man: time (i.e., when the Sabbath begins or ends)